Practical Dental Anaesthesia

Other Churchill Livingstone Dental Books

Practical Dental Anaesthesia

A. Kilpatrick

B.A.(Hons)., L.R.C.P. & S.(Edin)., L.R.F.P.S.G.,
D.A., D.R.C.O.G.
CONSULTANT ANAESTHETIST
LANCASTER DISTRICT HOSPITALS

CHURCHILL LIVINGSTONE
EDINBURGH LONDON AND NEW YORK 1979

CHURCHILL LIVINGSTONE
Medical Division of the Longman Group Limited

Distributed in the United States of America by Churchill
Livingstone Inc., 19 West 44th Street, New York,
N.Y. 10036, and by associated companies, branches and
representatives throughout the world.

First published 1979

ISBN 0 443 02076 0

British Library Cataloguing in Publication Data
Kilpatrick, A
 Practical dental anaesthesia.
 1. Anaesthesia in dentistry
I. Title
 617'.967'6   RK510   79-40315

Printed in Great Britain by T. & A. Constable Ltd., Edinburgh.

Preface

First of all it must be stated that this is not intended to be a completely comprehensive guide to out-patient dental anaesthesia. It is felt, however, that a considerable experience of the subject spanning a period of twenty years, ought to be able to offer some useful thoughts to others. It is envisaged that these 'others' fall into three categories. Firstly, dental students should be interested in a strictly practical guide to a subject which will be with them throughout their careers, either as operator or as anaesthetist. Secondly, junior anaesthetists who, as a rule, do not receive much practical instruction or experience of the subject, may find the book of practical use as it describes a system which is found to work satisfactorily and has been developed over a long period of time. They could perhaps adopt these techniques as they start in dental anaesthetic practice, prepared to modify the methods later, in the light of their own experience. Thirdly, established dental anaesthetists may be able to use some techniques or points as food for thought as they examine their own working methods. It is hoped they will pick up an occasional useful point of view as the author is sure he would, if examining their methods. There is a brief account of the costs involved — anaesthetic drugs and apparatus — which should be of interest to those about to embark upon a career as a dental anaesthetist. It is, of course, well appreciated by the author that quoted costs and fees can quickly become outdated because of escalating drug costs and an annual review of fees but this risk has been accepted in the hope that, even though on the publication date these figures will be somewhat obsolete, they will give some indication of capital costs and running costs and their relationship to anaesthetic fees.

The author wishes to acknowledge gratefully the help he received from Mr Philip Harrison, Senior Medical Photographer of the Royal Lancaster Infirmary, who prepared all the illustrations.

Lancaster, 1979   A.K.

Contents

1

Introduction

Over the past twenty years or more the author has become increasingly aware of a changing pattern in out-patient dental anaesthesia. In his earliest experience, the greater proportion of the anaesthetic sessions was occupied by patients attending for dental clearances. At this time, in one practice alone, where virtually the only anaesthetics given by the author were for major clearances, the number of patients awaiting an appointment for these sessions amounted to at least thirty. Nowadays, in this same practice, instead of dealing with five clearances at a session it is rare to exceed two and there is virtually no waiting period. In other practices only a small proportion of patients attend for dental clearances or part clearances. Following the years when clearances were common, there occurred a period when the major part of each session was devoted to children. Now, as the dental health of children has improved, only about 40 per cent of patients are 14 years of age or younger: the rest are adults. Less than 10 per cent are for clearances or part clearances, the other 90 per cent having less than six teeth extracted. It has proved of great interest to watch this changing pattern of treatment which has reflected the considerable improvement in dental health in both children and adults over this 23-year period.

When one considers the currently fashionable term, 'job satisfaction', in relation to dental anaesthesia, one finds that this exists in surprisingly generous proportions. The contact with the patient is admittedly brief, but in that short space of time the anaesthetist has the opportunity to establish a rapport with the patient by engaging in conversation, probably biased towards elucidating any doubtful aspects of his or her medical history, but at the same time creating confidence in the patient. This trust is important because a high proportion of patients, adults as well as children, return for further extractions at a later date, and if confidence is established at the first visit it is usually maintained. If one can successfully establish an air of quiet confidence and calm with the patient and a trust which is carried over to subsequent visits, the dental anaesthetist can claim to have attained a degree of job satisfaction.

Anaesthesia for out-patient dental surgery requires a more special working relationship between surgeon and anaesthetist than almost any other type of surgery. Any general surgeon and anaesthetist can co-operate together to operate on a hernia, varicose veins or almost any minor or routine major operation without previous experience of each other's working methods and without difficulties arising. This certainly does not apply to out-patient dental anaesthesia. The dental surgeon and the anaesthetist must be familiar with each other's techniques and the anaesthetist particularly must be aware at all times of how the surgery is progressing. Before the induction he must know how many and which teeth are to be extracted. If there is any history of difficult extractions the anaesthetist should have this information. During the procedure, because the anaesthetist is firmly holding the patient's head and providing counter-pressure to oppose the push of the dental forceps down the roots of the tooth, he becomes aware, at the same time as the dentist, of the early stages of the loosening of each tooth. The anaesthetist becomes aware when difficulties arise— teeth may be more firmly held in their sockets than normally; occasionally roots or apices may break off and be retained requiring a prolongation of the anaesthetic to remove them; bleeding may be more copious than usual, perhaps because of known inflammatory disease of the gums.

Furthermore, the dental anaesthetist must not be averse to lending a hand in the surgery whether it is to tidy the working surfaces before the next patient enters the room, to prepare mouth washes or to do anything else which is required. It is in the anaesthetist's own interests to speed up the changeover from one patient to the next.

There is too, a special relationship between patient and anaesthetist. The patient is aware, much more than he is in hospital, of who is administering his anaesthetic. The anaesthetist may be known to the patient through previous attention to himself or to his family or even his friends and this relationship plays a very important role in the building up of confidence in the patient. The patient may appear in the surgery for extractions in a very apprehensive frame of mind, an attitude initiated by a fear of dental treatment of any kind, perhaps caused by an unfortunate experience many years before or because of 'horror stories' told by one child to another. Except in exceptional circumstances, the patient is unpremedicated, and will have abstained from eating or drinking for several hours, which serves to remind him of the ordeal he is about to face. Most anaesthetists would describe the unpremedicated out-patient for general anaesthesia as one of the most difficult patients with whom one has to deal. The apprehensive patient with no experience, personal or vicarious, is probably the most difficult patient — and usually the most impressed afterwards when he wakes up and realizes how atraumatic the experience has been. Fortunately most dental patients are young and fit and present no problems from the point of view of general health. Those who do present problems due to health, or drugs which they regularly take, are almost always discovered by the dentist's questioning at an earlier visit or from information volunteered by the patient as a result of an instructive leaflet given to all patients attending for general anaesthesia. Nevertheless, the anaesthetist, prior to induction, still has time to question the patient to reveal relevant disabilities such as shortness of breath, anginal pains and so on. However, by far the commonest complaint is fear.

In contrast to the apprehensive patient, the casual patient presents an entirely different set of problems. He often disregards instructions given beforehand. He may come unaccompanied by an adult to see him home afterwards, often stating that he has no one who could attend at the appropriate time. One is often suspicious of these statements, believing the lack of a companion to be due principally to lack of effort on the patient's part to find someone. This creates the problem of whether or not to anaesthetise them. It is unadvisable to do so for several reasons. Firstly, their safety on the way home, when their reactions may be slightly dulled, will be at risk. Secondly, the anaesthetist's responsibility to the patient cannot be exercised fully and thirdly, the patient may continue to ignore this and other instructions on a future occasion. In the same way, some patients, otherwise responsible citizens, will ignore instructions not to drive their cars until the next day and, instead, drive to the surgery with every intention of driving home afterwards. The casual approach can often be put down to an irresponsible attitude to life in general but can just as often be attributed to a lack of understanding of the procedure and its implications — thinking that, for example, dental extractions are not really an 'operation', even though more blood is often spilled than in an appendicectomy or hernia repair, or that the anaesthetic is so 'light' and of such short duration that it can be discounted. This all adds up to a description of one of the hazards facing the dental anaesthetist, for a quick assessment of the patient's attitude and possible apprehensions must be made in the minute or two he is in the operating room prior to the induction of anaesthesia.

It is not generally appreciated by the anaesthetist who has no experience of anaesthesia in the dental chair that there is a considerable amount of physical effort required. The anaesthetist must provide counter-pressure against the push of the dental forceps and his fingers and forearms must take the strain when lower teeth are being extracted. When possible — and it is not always possible with some modern dental chairs — counter-pressure for upper extractions is provided by the anaesthetist's chest wall. In some modern fixed back chairs the upward pressure can only be resisted by the anaesthetist's arms and his firm grip of the patient's head. In addition the anaesthetist may be required to steady the head against lateral movements as the dentist breaks down the lingual or buccal plates in preparation for the extraction. If the anaesthetist is satisfactorily accomplishing his various duties in maintaining the patient's airway, by resisting manoeuvres of the dental surgeon which may obstruct the airway and at the same time providing counter-pressure during the efforts to extract the teeth, he will find that a long dental anaesthetic session will be physically demanding and tiring, resulting in aching shoulders and arm muscles until these muscles have become attuned to the unaccustomed exercise.

Consideration must be given to the special problems associated with anaesthetising the patient in the sitting position. Much has been written about this in the past (Bourne, 1957) but the dental anaesthetist is left with a problem for which there is no entirely satisfactory answer. If the patient is kept sitting upright with the legs in the normal dependent position, there must be an increased risk of hypotension occurring during the administration. However, if the chair back is lowered so that the patient is in a supine position, there must be an increased risk (in spite of throat packs) of foreign material — blood, filling material or broken pieces of tooth — dropping back towards the pharynx and larynx. This opinion is supported in an important recent article by Al-Khishali et al. (1978) who state that 'the horizontal position would appear to offer no obvious advantages in terms of the ease of maintenance of a patent airway, nor more likely to guarantee less soiling of the tracheo–bronchial tree with foreign material'. This horizontal position is further complicated by the fact that, at the end of the administration, the pack has to be removed, or at least partly removed, during the recovery period and, at this stage, the author believes the supine position to be positively dangerous. He has reached a compromise which, in his experience, proves satisfactory and adopts for the patient a position midway between upright and supine for the induction and maintenance of anaesthesia. There is at the same time a strong preference for a dental chair which has a leg support, continuous with the chair seat, which keeps the legs level with the pelvis. These chairs can tilt this leg support up slightly so that the feet are higher than the pelvis and this position is preferred. As soon as the administration is discontinued, the patient's body is tipped forward and his neck slightly flexed so that his mouth is tilted downwards, causing any free blood to flow out of the mouth and not back towards the larynx. It is difficult to see how this manoeuvre can be as satisfactorily and quickly carried out from a supine position. It must be remembered by the dental anaesthetist working in several dental practices that while he will have firm views on the ideal conditions for the patient and the anaesthetist, he must make the best use of the equipment available to him at the various surgeries, provided he is satisfied the patient is not endangered. Dental chairs, for example, are very expensive items of furniture and dental surgeons cannot reasonably be expected to spend £1000 or so on a new chair to replace one which will do almost as well. What ought to occur is that whenever the purchase of a new chair is contemplated the anaesthetist should be involved in the choice of the new chair. Meanwhile the anaesthetist must make the best use of whatever equipment is available to him by adapting his techniques to suit, unless the equipment is hopelessly outdated or dangerous.

While on the subject of equipment, and dental chairs in particular, it must be pointed out that the anaesthetist's first duty on commencing work in an unfamiliar surgery must be to familiarise himself with the equipment, especially the chair. There are a variety of methods for raising, lowering or tilting chairs and with these the anaesthetist must be expert. Should the need arise to tilt the chair head down, for example, this must be accomplished without a moment wasted in thought or a search for release levers.

Finally, a word about speed. As the reader will be aware, dental surgeons and anaesthetists, are paid on an 'item-of-service' basis. If for no other reason, time must not be wasted. By advocating this it does not mean patients should be rushed unduly or that safety should be endangered; however, it does mean that, consistent with safety (which is paramount) the anaesthetics should be administered expeditiously. Probably the dentist has allocated an hour or some other unit of time to his general anaesthetic session and all the patients sent for this session have to be attended to. Also, the anaesthetist may have an appointment at another place immediately afterwards and it is consequently in his interests not to waste time. In the author's experience patients can be anaesthetised in a civilised manner at a rate of six patients in an hour if one surgery and recovery room are used. If more than one surgery is used and there is plenty of ancillary help available, slightly more patients can be dealt with within this time by transferring the anaesthetic equipment from one surgery to another. However, it cannot be repeated too often that safe anaesthesia is the most important factor in dental anaesthesia. If this can be done expeditiously so much the better.

2

Gaseous induction and maintenance of anaesthesia

This procedure is used principally for young children under the age of fourteen years. This arbitrary age limit is only loosely applied because children younger than fourteen years will occasionally request an intravenous induction, often prompted to do so by a parent. However, the younger the child, the more likely is he to be frightened by injections and a sympathetically administered gaseous induction is usually more acceptable. A further drawback to the use of intravenous injections in children is that they can have a longer recovery period than adults and this delay in recovery of consciousness is often not acceptable to the parents who may worry that all is not well if their child does not recover as quickly as a child given a gaseous induction, even though they are assured that the delayed recovery period is regarded as normal. In practice they are warned of this beforehand.

As regards the gaseous induction, it is believed that the anaesthetist's approach to the patient is of extreme importance. He must chat to the child to interest him in something other than the anaesthetic. The subject of the conversation must be aimed at finding out something of interest to the child and obtaining a response in the form of an interested reply. The anaesthetist should be conversant with the recent activities in the football scene, the recent results of leading clubs, forthcoming international matches and so on as this is a ready source of conversation with boys. The girls are more interested in fashions, dolls, holiday activities and, occasionally, even boyfriends and these subjects can usually provide a conversational topic for the necessary few minutes. Some children respond to gentle teasing or leg-pulling and this is enough to distract their attention. The important point here is that the child's attention must be held.

While all this talk is proceeding the anaesthetist must be able to incorporate instructions into the conversation and also an explanation of what he is doing. The author prefers the child to sit, leaning back against the upright part of the chair, with the head resting on the support and the hands clasped gently on the lap — clasped hands with the fingers interlaced are often difficult to unclasp during uncoordinated movements (should they occur under general anaesthesia) thus keeping the patient's hands away from the anaesthetic equipment during induction. It will be remembered that while anaesthesia deepens the various stages of anaesthesia are passed through, as described by Guedel (1951), and the same stages are passed through during recovery from anaesthesia. As the child passes through the stage of excitement both during induction and recovery, uncoordinated confused movements may occur, though they are commoner during the recovery period. It is always advisable to extinguish the operating light during the induction and recovery phases as this bright light shining on the patient's eyes, even when closed, can aggravate any tendency to restlessness. Having suitably adjusted the chair and head rest and persuaded the child to clasp his hands, a nasal mask held in a cupped right hand is placed in front of the face, the ulnar edge of the hand resting gently on the patient's chin and the mask resting on the uppermost part of the hand and held in place by the thumb. The mask should be two or three inches from the face, the cupped hand enlarging the effective size of the mask and forming a reservoir from which the patient breathes the gas mixture being delivered. During this manoeuvre the child must be told what is being done, and he is asked to listen for the gentle wind which will flow over his face. He is told, too, that this wind will, in a minute or two, make him feel sleepy and that his feet will begin to tingle. The author believes it is also wise to suggest to the child that he will have a

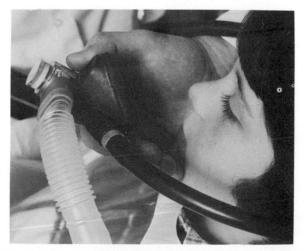

Fig. 2.1 This illustrates the full use of the right hand in enlarging the effective size of the mask while holding the mask far enough away from the patient's face not to cause discomfort. The East scavenging valve is illustrated.

pleasant dream, even to suggest a subject for that dream — for example, Christmas activities, summer holidays or whatever else is seasonal or appropriate at the time. As the child is recovering he can often be persuaded that he has dreamed about the chosen subject — getting in first with a suggestion of a pleasant experience or dream is better than waiting for the child to tell the anaesthetist that he has had an unpleasant dream. While the induction is proceeding there must be silence in the surgery apart from the conversation of the anaesthetist.

The gas flow should be high and in some types of apparatus there is no alternative to a high flow rate. Some machines, notably the McKesson Simplor machines, do not allow an accurate estimation of the gas flow and it is left, in these circumstances, to the anaesthetist to assess the flow requirements from the sound of the gas flow, the rate at which the reservoir bag fills and a familiarity with the particular apparatus. The mixture of gases recommended is nitrous oxide with 25 per cent oxygen and this is left unchanged throughout the administration. Higher percentages of oxygen result in a longer induction period and lower percentages are unjustified in that they tend towards oxygen deprivation. While the gases are flowing and the conversation with the patient is proceeding as described above, halothane vapour is introduced into the circuit, slowly at first, after the child has taken 10–15 breaths of the gaseous mixture, and then fairly rapidly. When the maximum halothane concentration to be delivered — usually 3 per cent on graduated vaporisers is sufficient — has proved acceptable to the patient it is usually safe to place the mask over the nose in contact with the face to make a firm gas-tight seal. Expired gases are then expelled through a freely opened expiratory valve, preferably attached to a scavenging device. The patient's mouth may now be opened by means of a gag which is placed between the teeth on the opposite side of the jaws to the side to be operated upon. The jaws will have relaxed sufficiently for the gag to be placed in position and for the mouth to be opened readily. If this cannot be done, insufficient anaesthesia has been obtained and the administration is continued until a gag can be inserted and the mouth opened. Once the mouth is open the anaesthetist must assess the anaesthetic requirements in terms of the number of extractions to be carried out and whether they may be expected to be accomplished easily or not. In practice this means that if only 1 or 2 deciduous teeth have to be extracted, the halothane may be discontinued immediately the gag and pack are in place. If several teeth have to be extracted — for example 4 first molars — the halothane is first reduced to half its induction concentration when the mouth is opened and packed and then discontinued when half the extractions are completed.

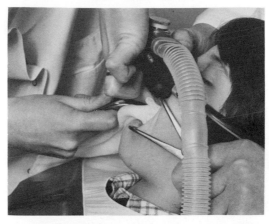

Fig. 2.2 The picture shows the anaesthetist controlling the nasal mask with his right hand and the Ferguson gag with the left while an upper right tooth is being extracted. Counter pressure is exerted by the use of the anaesthetist's chest on the top of the child's head.

When the extractions are completed, the gas flow is discontinued immediately, the mask removed from the face and the gag removed from the mouth. The pack placed in the mouth by the dentist prior to the extractions is either left in position with a 'tail' hanging out of the mouth sufficient to give the anaesthetist a firm grip of it or, if there is any suggestion at all that it may obstruct the airway, it is pulled a little way out of the mouth leaving sufficient gauze in the mouth to absorb any blood oozing from the sockets. At the conclusion of the operation the pack must be unequivocally the responsibility of the anaesthetist. He must be the one to decide when to ease it forward or remove it and he should do this himself. The head is held forwards with the body upright or leaning forwards, with the mouth inclined towards the floor to encourage any blood not absorbed by the pack to trickle out of the mouth and not backwards towards the larynx. The child should soon begin to show signs of regaining consciousness — restless movements, opening his eyes, responding to instructions to push the pack out of his mouth and then to spit into a bowl held in front of his chin. During recovery of consciousness the patient is best left undisturbed as too early stimulation can precipitate restlessness and struggling. If it is thought that consciousness has been regained but that the patient is simply just sitting with his eyes shut, it is in order to speak sharply to the patient encouraging him to spit in the bowl and to open his eyes, or even to use a painful stimulus — squeezing the trapezius muscle or pressing firmly on the posterior edge of the ramus of the mandible. However, too early use of a painful stimulus can

B

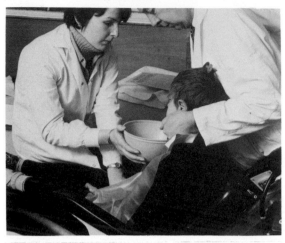

Fig. 2.3 The patient's body has been pushed forwards while his head is securely held, airway is maintained and the head tilted slightly towards the floor to allow blood to trickle out into the bowl rather than backwards towards the larynx and trachea.

cause increased restlessness. Once the child has opened his eyes, can keep them open and responds to conversation and instructions he can either be walked to a nearby recovery room or the anaesthetist may move his apparatus to an adjacent surgery to attend to the next patient. The child will require 5 or 10 minutes more to recover sufficiently to be allowed home in the care of a responsible adult.

During the administration one must pay strict attention to the patient's airway and this is not always easy. The mouth is propped open either by the use of a gag — the Ferguson and Doyen types are the most commonly used — or a dental prop — either the rubber McKesson side props or a spring-loaded centre prop. The gag may be inserted after the patient has been anaesthetised but props are more often placed in position prior to induction. When the patient is unconscious and the mouth has been opened, the dentist places a pack in the mouth behind the level of the teeth to be extracted to prevent blood and tooth fragments from passing backwards towards the larynx and this also discourages the patient from mouth breathing during anaesthesia. Should the patient breathe through his mouth around the pack during the administration, control of his level of unconsciousness is lost and an unsatisfactory anaesthetic results with the patient's depth of anaesthesia becoming too light and restless movements consequently taking place. Although in the author's experience the most commonly used packing material is a length of dental gamgee cut from a roll, the important issue here is not the type of pack used but the care with which it is placed in position. A badly placed pack can ruin an anaesthetic by either causing obstruction to the airway or by enabling intake of air via the mouth, leading to dilution of the anaesthetic gases delivered to the patient and an uncontrolled anaesthetic. While the pack is placed in position by the dentist, the wishes of the anaesthetist in this matter must be heeded for, as stated, a malpositioned pack can prevent smooth anaesthesia. This is one of the areas in which familiarity, on the part of the anaesthetist, with the working methods and ability of the surgeon is important because some dentists are, unfortunately, not quite as expert at inserting a mouth pack as others.

The position of the patient in the dental chair is very important but in advising on this situation one has first of all to make the best use of the available chairs. A variety of chairs will be encountered and most chairs will have advantages and disadvantages from the point of view of the anaesthetist. We, as anaesthetists have preferences and ought to be consulted when a new chair is being purchased, but we must remember that these chairs are being used for conservative dentistry for 38 or 39 hours a week against the one or two hours when they are used for general anaesthesia. Modern dental chairs have a single portion for the patient to sit upon with his legs extended at the knees and resting on the supporting extension. This raising of the legs has the advantage that during anaesthesia there is less likelihood of blood to 'pool' in the legs. In old chairs, where the legs are not supported in this way, the writer prefers the knees to be bent and the heels pulled back to maintain a more stable position. However, while the seats of the modern chairs have advantages, the upright rigid back support has disadvantages. The upper part of the back may detach to allow the anaesthetist to reach over to attend to small children more easily. However, for adults the top is usually fixed in line with the chair back with only a small pad which may be placed behind the head or neck. Some patients have their thoracic spines so curved that in order to rest their heads on the support the head is thrown back at an unsatisfactory hyperextended angle. A variety of small boxes can be kept handy to place between the head cushion and the chair back in order to keep the patient's head in a comfortable position suitable for general anaesthesia.

The angle of the chair back is important and this is to some extent controversial. The author prefers the back to be semi-reclining with the whole chair tipped back slightly but one must reach a compromise between the position most favourable in the event of hypotension occurring and the position in which foreign material in the mouth, such as blood, is least likely to fall or trickle into the pharynx and on to the larynx. Most chairs, especially the modern ones, allow this

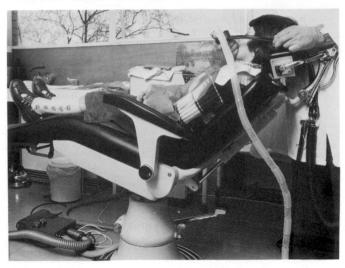

Fig. 2.4 The chair back is mid-way between fully erect and fully reclining with the seat tipped slightly back. This chair is used mainly for children and has a low back with a head piece which can be freely manipulated to suit each patient.

position to be obtained. Most modern chairs are electrically operated and the anaesthetist must familiarise himself with the controls. Whatever type of chair is being used the anaesthetist must know how to level the chair rapidly and without hesitation in the event of a hypotensive episode. As soon as the operation is completed it is essential to bring the patient's body into an upright position with his head forward and his mouth inclined towards the floor as described above. If the patient were anaesthetised in a fully reclining position it would be unwise to raise him abruptly to an upright position for fear of disturbing a temporarily unstable cardiovascular system. However, the only other safe procedure would be to turn him on his side — an impossible task in most chairs — and placing him at the risk of falling out of the chair. In spite of warnings of fainting in the dental chair during general anaesthesia the author prefers to use the semi-reclining position described above.

The question of fainting in the dental chair must be mentioned further, for some people will faint in the chair without anything being done to them at all. A faint during induction or maintenance must be watched for constantly and any suggestion of pallor or deterioration of the pulse must be treated by immediate levelling of the chair with the administration of high concentrations of oxygen with the use of intermittent positive pressure ventilation by manual compression of the reservoir bag, if necessary. This emergency treatment must take precedence, of course, over any operative procedure. Long experience in dental anaesthesia has not found fainting to occur often at all but its very infrequency only makes it all the more important for the anaesthetist to be on the look out constantly for its occurrence. While it is advisable and possible for the anaesthetist to keep a finger on an accessible pulse during a gaseous induction it unfortunately becomes a practical impossibility to do so during the hurly burly of the extraction procedure when the anaesthetist's hands are fully occupied steadying the patient's head, holding the nasal mask, holding the gag in place and freeing a hand occasionally when required to adjust the halothane concentration control.

During gaseous induction and maintenance it is believed the use of a reservoir bag in the circuit is important in order to demonstrate that an adequate tidal volume is being maintained. Formerly many dental anaesthetists just used a high flow of gases with no suggestion of re-breathing and without such a bag in the circuit. Others used a demand flow technique with gases only flowing on inspiration. The writer believes it is much wiser to be able to demonstrate to one's self that the patient is breathing freely using the gases from the anaesthetic apparatus.

Vomiting is a complication at the end of an anaesthetic administration and occurs more often following a gaseous induction than with intravenous inductions. In the author's experience this vomiting occurs mainly in the child who has been very apprehensive or frightened and has worked himself into a state of near panic prior to the induction. Previous experience of general anaesthesia followed by vomiting almost always maintains the sequence and vomiting occurs each time. It is suggested that previous experience of this kind is sufficient grounds for an intravenous induction on subsequent occasions if the child will allow it. The calm child very rarely vomits irrespective of the method of induction.

Finally one must discuss hands. The anaesthetist has only two of these like everyone else but to perform dental anaesthesia he has to use these to their utmost to do three or four things at the same time. During induction the cupped right hand is used to enlarge the effective size of the nasal mask while the left hand manipulates the gas and vapour controls. When the mask makes contact with the patient's face, the anaesthetist must be able to hold the mask in position, open the mouth gag and then steady it in position and, at the same time, steady the patient's head, provide counter pressure against the push of the forceps and be ready to free the left hand to manipulate the controls on the vaporiser and anaesthetic machine. Finally, at the conclusion of the anaesthetic the mask must be removed and hooked on to the back of the dental chair or anaesthetic machine, the patient's head controlled, the airway maintained and the gases switched off to avoid waste of expensive gases and unnecessary pollution of the atmosphere in the room. It is at times like these that the trainee dental anaesthetist often wishes he has more than one pair of hands.

3

Intravenous induction

Intravenous induction is used for all patients over 14 years of age, except on the few occasions when a gaseous induction is requested, and occasionally in younger children when specially requested or indicated. Special indications for use in younger children include a repeated history of vomiting after previous gaseous induction or an extreme fear of gaseous induction provided this fear does not extend also to a fear of injections. Any attempt to force an intravenous injection on an unwilling child is discouraged as it may make further visits even more traumatic and is very difficult, with a high risk of extravenous injection. In the early days of the use of methohexitone, an intramuscular injection of the drug was recommended to calm the child but the author did not accept this view and has not seen it recommended for many years. Diazepam, orally or by injection, an hour or more prior to the visit to the surgery would be more humane for the very reluctant child.

The author's personal choice of induction agent is methohexitone, being reliable, predictable, easy to use and convenient to carry about from surgery to surgery. Instead of the more generally recommended 1 per cent solution, a 2.5 per cent solution is used — 100 ml of sterile water in a large 2.5 g multidose bottle. To administer the drug 5 ml syringes are used which, being small, are more convenient to carry around than the large 20 ml syringes which would be required for the more usual 1 per cent solution. When mixing the drug 5 ml of 2 per cent lignocaine is added to the bottle of methohexitone because it is found that occasionally the intravenous injection of methohexitone — 1 per cent as well as the 2.5 per cent solution — is painful. The author is convinced that this small amount of lignocaine reduces the frequency of this pain. The other measure used to counter this discomfort is to inject the methohexitone into the larger veins of the antecubital fossa in preference to the veins on the back of the hand. The blood flow is brisker at the elbow and the drug is diluted more quickly by the greater volume of blood. It is prudent when injecting the barbiturate into the vein, to inject first a small amount, say one millilitre of the solution, and then enquire whether or not this has caused discomfort or actual pain, just as one would do if injecting thiopentone. The methohexitone, though not as irritating as thiopentone, would probably cause spasm of the artery if injected intra-arterially with the attendant possible risk of a peripherally gangrenous limb. The author has not for a long time used the oily-based intravenous agents as he has developed a personal prejudice against injecting the oil, largely because of the reports of cardio-vascular collapse following its use. There has even been a warning notice from the Committee on Safety of Medicines (February, 1978) telling of a syndrome associated with the administration of Althesin. This has taken the form of hypotension, bronchospasm and flushing which can occur, or possibly recur, after an interval of twelve hours or more. The single dose ampoules associated with these oily-based drugs are less convenient than the large multidose bottle of the water soluble methohexitone, whose dose can be estimated when the patient is examined and the required dose of the drug withdrawn into the syringe. In recent years the use of multidose bottles of drugs was discouraged but their use seems to be creeping back into fashion again. The author believes that when one person is carrying out the mixing of the drug and the water and he alone, infrequently and with great care, is placing sterile needles through the rubber cap of the bottle, no harm results. In estimating the dose of methohexitone, the author works on a basic 10 mg per stone (6 kg) of body weight but uses discretion in increasing this dose because of other factors such as temperament, extreme nervousness, alcoholic tolerance and habits, and even tattooing — for which he may add 12.5–25 mg of methohexitone. A maximum dose of 150 mg is used, which can be attained by overfilling the 5 ml syringe with an extra millilitre, thus putting 6 ml of the methohexitone in the syringe. The act of overfilling the 5 ml syringe with an extra millilitre does not prevent the routine aspiration of blood to confirm the correct location of the needle within the vein thus avoiding the hazards of an extravascular injection of an irritant drug. The observation on tattooing is explained by using the tattoo as an indication, particularly in the young adult, of an immaturity and emotional instability often associated with alcoholic excess. Old age warrants a considerable reduction in the basic dose. However, one hesitates to attribute this to 'old age', and therefore the writer begins to reduce the weight-related estimation after the age of 45 to 50. This is attributed to a more stable temperament in later middle age! It is very important, for medico-legal reasons as well as for assistance at a return visit to the surgery sometime in the future, to record the dosage of methohexitone required by the patient. Sometimes, it is found more practicable to record the optimum dose for that particular patient in the light of his reaction to the dose given rather than the actual dose administered. If, however, there is a significant difference between the dose administered and the estimated optimum dose — of say, 25 mg or more — then both figures are recorded. For example, should 100 mg be given and found satisfactory, that dose is recorded; but, if it is found to be inadequate and a dose of 125 mg, might have been more appropriate, then this dose is recorded too. Similarly if it were felt that a delay of recovery was due to a relative over dosage, then an estimated smaller dose is recorded as well as the one actually administered. It is also noted in the record if a halothane supplement was required because nitrous oxide and oxygen alone did not provide satisfactory operating conditions. Normally, having given an induction dose of methohexitone it is found that no supplement other than nitrous oxide and 25 per cent oxygen is required but this will depend upon an assessment of the amount of surgical work to be done and its nature and also upon the patient's response to the estimated induction dose — if this proves inadequate a supplement of halothane will certainly be required. If the methohexitone is injected quickly — and this is too easy to do using the more concentrated solution — brief respiratory depression and even apnoea may occur. The nasal mask, with the gases flowing, is placed over the patient's nose as soon as the injection is completed, the mandible is held forward to maintain an open airway and the head is held firmly between the anaesthetist's hands while holding a Ferguson or other gag in place with the patient's mouth opened. To relieve the respiratory depression, if it occurs, and in any case to achieve a smooth transition to the satisfactory maintenance of general anaesthesia, the author believes in the stimulating effect of early operative intervention. As soon as the mask, with the gases flowing, is in position and the mouth opened, a pack is positioned and extractions should begin. Some of the extractions are no doubt performed solely under the influence of the methohexitone. Depending upon the number of teeth to be extracted, the anaesthetist may find that a halothane supplement is required. Assessment on this point is made upon the patient's reaction. Should he show signs of becoming too lightly anaesthetised — involuntary movements of hands, arms or legs or phonation — halothane should be added and may usually be discontinued when three or four teeth of a clearance or part clearance remain to be extracted. This seems a suitable moment to point out that it is very important that the anaesthetist should know before the induction, just how many teeth have to be extracted and any other relevant information such as a history of difficult extractions, which might lead one to expect a prolonged anaesthetic.

It should really go without saying that strict attention to the airway is of paramount importance during the administration. If the airway is neglected or obstructed for any reason, the patient is in danger and the defect must be remedied immediately. A common cause of obstructed airway can be the mouth pack pushed too far back in the mouth or perhaps depressing the tongue. The operator's fingers can even cause obstruction as, for example, when a finger of his left hand is placed on the floor of the mouth in the lingual side of the teeth during the extraction of lower left molars. A patient's obesity can be the cause of obstruction and the writer well remembers a grossly obese, bullnecked man whose airway could not be maintained until a nasopharyngeal tube had been passed. These tubes are so invaluable in the presence of upper respiratory obstruction that the dental anaesthetist is strongly recommended to carry one or two in his pocket readily available whenever he is working.

Recovery following methohexitone induction is found to be quick, especially if halothane has not been required as a supplement. Often, the patient at the end of the operative procedure, sits contentedly in the chair with his eyes closed and only requires to be spoken to gently for him to turn, when requested, to the basin at his side, to spit out, and then rinse his mouth. The patient is often found to be sitting quietly waiting for the procedure to begin — he wakes up astonished to find that the extractions have been completed. The mouth pack is partly removed from the mouth at the end of the extractions but a

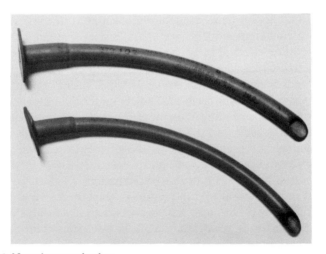

Fig. 3.1 Nasopharyngeal tubes

portion of it should remain in the mouth until the patient responds to the request to open his mouth and then spit out. While awaiting this moment the patient is sitting upright with his head held forwards and slightly downwards so that blood not caught by the pack may flow out of the mouth rather than backwards towards the pharynx and larynx. It is the practice of some dental surgeons to insert the patient's new dentures in cases of dental clearances, before consciousness has been regained. Blood is cleared from the mouth by mopping with a pack or suction or both and the dentures are placed in position. Provided this is done carefully, without squeezing blood backwards behind the dentures, this practice does reduce the amount of immediate postoperative haemorrhage because of the pressure exerted by the dentures.

4

Endotracheal intubation for O.P. dental procedures

It is only right and proper that a warning should begin this chapter. The techniques described are only to be considered by doctors who have successfully undergone a prolonged period of formal anaesthetic training. Endotracheal intubation cannot be contemplated by anyone without this training, adequate equipment and preferably with trained assistants who are familiar with the equipment and the anaesthetist's method of working. It is not a procedure suitable for the 'occasional' anaesthetist and requires a certain minimum of equipment for safe intubation — laryngoscope with different sizes of blade and fresh batteries, Magill forceps, a supply of endotracheal tubes of different sizes with their connections, throat packs, suitable lubricants for the tubes and, of course, an anaesthetic machine capable of providing oxygen and nitrous oxide under controlled flow rates and a means of delivering an adjuvant such as halothane or trichlorethylene. The anaesthetic apparatus must be able to to be used to ventilate a paralysed patient. In addition an aspirator, of the high volume displacement type, must be readily available.

Endotracheal intubation is used in circumstances where some difficulty is anticipated either in the nature of the surgical problems or where some anaesthetic difficulty may be expected. These categories include the following:

1. History of difficult extractions where multiple extractions or a dental clearance is to be carried out.

2. 'Surgical' extractions of unerupted wisdom teeth or other unerupted teeth such as palatally buried canines.

3. Patients with multiple roots for extraction where the problem of searching for these roots can be difficult or impossible using a nasal mask technique because of blood obscuring vision or trickling towards the respiratory passages. Intubation allows a specially careful search for these roots helped by X-rays of the sites.

4. Alveolectomies where bone has to be carefully removed until the correct amount has been excised for cosmetic reasons.

5. Apicectomies.

6. Conservation work on extremely nervous patients, especially in children where many fillings have to be done over a period of perhaps an hour.

7. Anaesthetic considerations, the commonest occurring when it is anticipated that there will be difficulty in maintaining the airway using only a nasal mask. The most frequent cause of this difficulty is extreme obesity of the patient.

In June 1958 the author began to develop the following method of anaesthetising patients which has been found to work satisfactorily from the point of view of the patient, the surgeon and the anaesthetist. Anaesthesia is induced with the patient in the sitting position, semi-reclining, since we believe (especially in the early days of our experience) that patients are less alarmed and consequently more at ease by being dealt with in what they regard as the usual posture for dental treatment. In recent years, of course, many dental surgeons carry out conservative work with conscious patients in a supine position so the general public regards this reclining position with less alarm than formerly. Nevertheless we have continued to use the sitting position as we have found it to be safe for the patients and does not give them cause for undue concern.

Prior to induction, syringes are prepared containing thiopentone in a dose of between 250 mg and 400 mg, atropine 0.5 mg either in a separate 2 ml syringe or mixed with the thiopentone, and suxamethonium 70 mg in a 2 ml syringe. At this stage the anaesthetic machine and its cylinders have been checked as have the other items of equipment required to oxygenate the patient and then proceed to intubation. A 'cockpit drill' is recommended whereby the various stages of the procedure about to be followed are enacted in sequence in the anaesthetist's mind as he visually checks every item of equipment. The patient is seated comfortably in the chair with both sleeves rolled up to the elbow, clothing loosened around the neck and waist, a plastic bib tied loosely round his neck to protect his clothing from soiling and his head lying on a headrest which has been suitably adjusted. After applying a venous tourniquet, a needle is placed in a suitable vein, preferably on the dorsum of his hand to reduce the risk of intra-arterial injection. The atropine, if in a separate syringe, is injected first, followed by the thiopentone, the dose of which has been estimated beforehand taking into consideration the patient's sex, age, weight, the presence or otherwise of above average apprehension and, of course, his social habits— mainly alcohol consumption. Remember these are unpremedicated patients whose main cause for confidence in their medical and dental attendants is based on an understanding built up over years of attendance for regular treatment or upon the

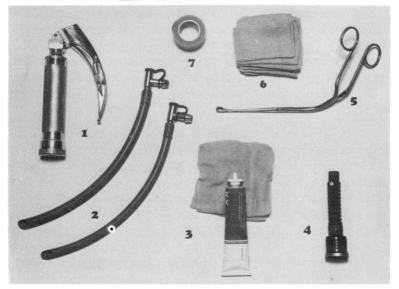

Fig. 4.1 Equipment which should be ready prior to induction of anaesthesia when the patient is to be intubated.

1. Macintosh laryngoscope
2. Magill nasotracheal tubes
3. KY Lubricant Jelly
4. Catheter mount
5. Magill forceps
6. Gauze throat pack
7. Clear Tape

reputation and standing of the practice in the town. In extreme cases of apprehension the patients may be calmed with a suitable dose of diazepam on the night before the operation and perhaps a repeat dose a few hours prior to the anaesthetic, but in the writer's experience this is rarely necessary and is best avoided as it will probably delay full recovery of consciousness. The author uses the patient's left hand for the injection with the dentist standing by the patient's left shoulder helping to support the arm and ready to move behind the chair to control the head should it fall forward, and with the nurse standing on the patient's right ready to control the patient's arms to prevent them falling towards the floor when he is laid flat but these positions can obviously be modified to suit the layout of other surgeries. As soon as the patient is unconscious, the suxamethonium is injected and the dentist immediately and rapidly manipulates the chair into a horizontal position while the anaesthetist moves to take control of the patient's head and airway. While the arms are being tied loosely together at the wrist by the dental nurse and the headrest is being adjusted by the dentist under the anaesthetist's guidance into the correct position to support the head in the ideal position for blind

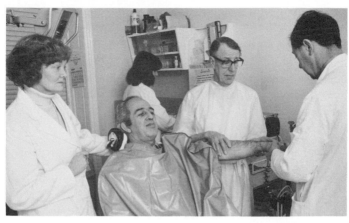

Fig. 4.2 The patient is seated comfortably in the normal sitting position, draped with a protective apron. The patient's arm is supported by the dentist while the intravenous injection is given. The chairside assistant stands by to assist and to take control of the patient's arms as soon as he is unconscious.

nasotracheal intubation, the anaesthetist is ventilating the patient's lungs with oxygen. This correct position is one where the neck is flexed in the cervico-thoracic region and extended in the upper cervical spine to give the impression that the patient is 'sniffing the morning air'.

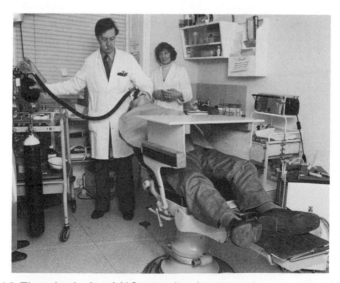

Fig. 4.3 The patient has been laid flat, arms have been secured to prevent them falling towards the floor, the headrest has been suitably adjusted and the patient's lungs are being ventilated with oxygen.

As soon as relaxation is complete, an already well-lubricated nasotracheal tube is inserted into the right nostril and passed through the nose and pharynx to the larynx where, if the head is positioned correctly the tube will in most cases pass through into the trachea. If the tube fails to pass at the first attempt it may be seen, by viewing the front of the neck, to protrude on either side of the larynx, most commonly on the right side. By withdrawing the tube slightly and

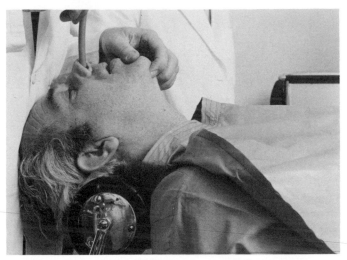

Fig. 4.4 This picture illustrates the flexion of the neck on the thoracic spine with the extension of the head on the neck. This tube passed straight through the larynx into the trachea at the first attempt.

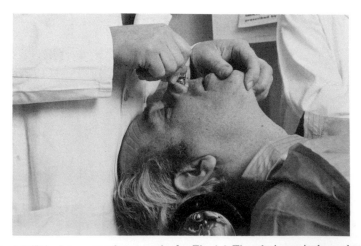

Fig. 4.5 This picture was taken seconds after Fig. 4.4. The tube is now in the trachea.

twisting it, by manipulating the connection, towards the mid-line, a second attempt may be successful, perhaps combined with the flexion of the neck which can be accomplished by the anaesthetist using his abdomen as a 'third hand' to aid the left hand to manoeuvre the head and flex the neck slightly. If this attempt fails it is not wise to persist with blind intubation but to resort to the insertion of a Macintosh laryngoscope (Fig. 4.1) and the placement of the tip of the tube between the vocal cords by using Magill forceps (Fig. 4.1). When the tube is in place it is connected immediately to a Boyle machine and

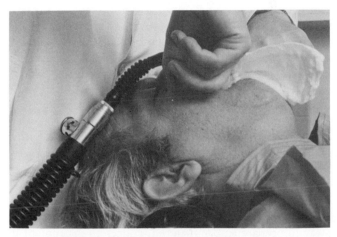

Fig. 4.6 The endotracheal tube has been connected to the Boyle apparatus and the lungs ventilated with oxygen again, before the pharyngeal pack is inserted using the index fingers of both hands.

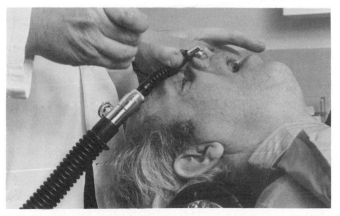

Fig. 4.7 The tube is securely fastened using non-reactive sticky tape, following which surgery may now begin.

C

ventilation is continued with nitrous oxide and oxygen with trichlorethylene vapour added. This ventilation is only interrupted to place, with great care, a gauze throat pack, moistened in water or saline, in the pharynx and fasten the tube in place with a length of adhesive non-reactive tape such as 'Cleartape' (Fig. 4.1). Apart from this brief interruption, ventilation is continued by manual compression of the reservoir bag until spontaneous respiration occurs again in a few minutes. The surgical procedure may commence as soon as the pack and adhesive tape are in position. Thereafter, anaesthesia continues smoothly until the operation is concluded. An important point to watch for is unwanted movements of the patient's head caused by the surgical manoeuvres which may precipitate coughing on the tube. This can usually be dealt with by steadying of the head, increasing the Trilene vapour strength or, in extreme cases, by small supplementary doses of thiopentone or even sux-amethonium. The other significant point, which should really not need to be mentioned, is to watch for disconnection in some point of the Magill anaesthetic circuit. In normal practice, the anaesthetist is able to assist the dental surgeon by steadying the head, providing counter-pressure with his hip or hands when upper teeth are being extracted and even wielding a surgical hammer when bone is being chiselled away to allow, for example, the removal of impacted wisdom teeth. It is also possible for the anaesthetist to relieve temporarily the dental assistant by manipulating the suction handpiece while she turns away to prepare suture material, collect an instrument from a sterilizer and so on. Briefly, while watching the patient carefully, the anaesthetist can easily make himself useful by helping the surgeon — after all there is not room for more people round the patient's head once the surgeon, anaesthetist, chairside assistant and the anaesthetic apparatus are in position.

Once the surgical procedure is completed Trilene is discontinued and the nitrous oxide–oxygen mixture is changed to 100 per cent oxygen, a recovery couch is wheeled alongside the chair, the arm of the chair on the same side is lowered, the chair is pumped up level with the recovery couch and the patient is lifted or pulled bodily on to the couch, taking care to avoid injury to the head and neck. In the same movement the patient is turned on his side. The pack is removed, an airway is inserted if the patient will tolerate it and the nasotracheal tube is removed. The patient is now wheeled to the recovery room through a communicating door, the couch is stabilized by fastening it to the wall, and a trained nurse cares for the patient and his airway until consciousness is regained. It is rare for the recovery period to last more than 30 minutes by the end of which time the

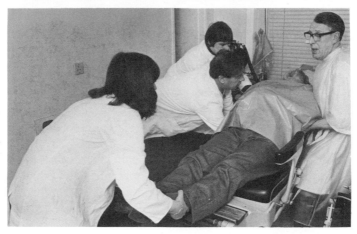

Fig. 4.8 Surgery completed, a trolley is wheeled alongside the chair, the arm on that side removed and the patient lifted on to the trolley while he is still connected to the anaesthetic machine. As he is lifted over the patient is turned on to his left side.

patient is usually fit to leave for home in a car or taxi accompanied by a responsible adult. Finally, instructions are given to the patient regarding his behaviour during the rest of that day — no driving of cars, no manipulation of machinery, no alcohol and so on.

As an alternative to the use of thiopentone for induction the author has many times used methohexitone — and this drug or one of the

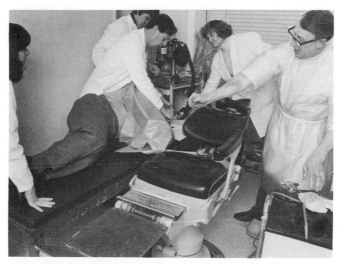

Fig. 4.9 The patient is now on his side and ready to have the pharyngeal pack and then the endotracheal tube removed. He is next wheeled to an adjacent recovery room in the care of a nurse.

other ultra short- acting induction agents may well appeal to other anaesthetists who may not accept that thiopentone can be used with such a rapid recovery time. It is felt that these short-acting drugs have too short an action for use with Trilene and consequently it is much more difficult to maintain smooth anaesthesia. Methohexitone is the writer's favourite drug among these short-acting induction agents largely because it is in a watery solution which is more easily injected intravenously and he readily admits a prejudice, previously stated, against the intravenous use of oily solutions because of the difficulty of injection but principally because of the reported cardiovascular collapses using oil-based preparations. If methohexitone or one of the other short-acting induction agents is used the anaesthetist will probably find that he requires to administer halothane rather than the less expensive Trilene for satisfactory maintenance of anaesthesia.

COMPLICATIONS AND DIFFICULTIES

The outstanding complication most to be feared when using suxamethonium on out-patients is obviously that of prolonged apnoea. In twenty years of using this technique this has happened only once. This required the anaesthetist to ventilate the patient for three hours at the end of which time she recovered and was transferred to the local hospital for an overnight stay. Investigations later found that this lady and her family had low serum cholinesterase levels and their names were added to the locally held register of such families. They were warned to point out their susceptability on future occasions when they required general anaesthetics. When a suxamethonium-induced prolonged apnoea does occur all the members of the patient's family as well as the patient himself must be tested for abnormally low serum cholinesterase levels and all those discovered to be deficient in this enzyme must be warned to declare this information should they ever require an anaesthetic in hospital or elsewhere.

Suxamethonium pains have not proved a significant hazard even though they have been sought. A few patients have mentioned to the dental surgeon at a subsequent visit that they have had an ache in the neck or chest postoperatively but in none has it proved disabling. Therefore, the author's attitude has been to ignore it for all practical purposes, though he is aware that occasionally a patient may be more inconvenienced by these suxamethonium pains than by the discomfort at the operation site. It is believed that the advantage to be gained by using suxamethonium greatly outweighs the disadvantages of these pains — and of the very occasional possibility of a prolonged apnoea.

Regurgitation during induction has never occurred and this has been credited to the fact that patients have obeyed strict instructions to have nothing to eat or drink in the four hours prior to induction. This is made easier for our patients by their being operated upon early, usually before 10 a.m., on a Saturday morning and so they are not exposed to the temptation to eat or drink for long before the anaesthesia. In practice they come to the surgery premises soon after rising in the morning.

Delay in recovery has not proved a problem. As said earlier, the great majority of patients are fit to leave with an escort within thirty minutes after the conclusion of the operation. As a curtained recovery room with individual recovery couches is used there is no pressure on the accommodation and, therefore, no pressure on the patients to depart earlier than they ought to do. Should a patient not be fit to leave as early as one would normally expect, it is simply a matter of retaining them under observation for a longer period. In practice, the most difficult patients to deal with postoperatively are the teenagers. They tend towards a restless, confused recovery which may also be a little longer than average for adults. Over the years the writer has tended towards inducing anaesthesia in the teenager with methohexitone rather than thiopentone and this has reduced the confused restless phase and also the the recovery time.

Occasionally nasotracheal intubations encounter problems. First of all one or both nasal passages may be obstructed. It is customary to intubate through the right nostril when possible as it is always supposed that the endotracheal tube with its diagonally sectioned end

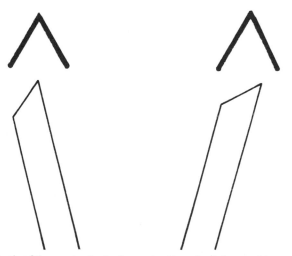

Fig. 4.10 The tip of the nasotracheal tube coming from the right nostril is more likely to reach the vocal chords in the mid-line than the tube coming from the left nostril.

lends itself to easier passage from the right nostril (Fig. 4.10). When the right side is too narrow to allow the passage of the tube time should not be wasted by persisting with fruitless attempts on the right side. If difficulty is encountered, switch attempts immediately to the left nostril which will be clear in the vast majority of instances. However, should this also be obstructed have no hesitation in passing the endotracheal tube orally. This may on rare occasions be inconvenient for some surgical manoeuvres but it is better for the patient and his safety to have an endotracheal tube passed, and passed without undue delay. Remember that the patient is apnoeic during all this time and that a quickly passed endotracheal tube — by any route — is essential if hypoxia is to be avoided. If there is any delay at all, ventilation with an oxygen rich mixture of gases should be carried out between attempts at intubation.

Difficulty may be induced by producing haemorrhage from the nasal passage due to trauma caused by the tube. This, when it occurs, has always been of minor significance but it could be profuse leading to the field of vision being obscured when using the laryngoscope (Fig. 4.1) or, even more important, to the entry of blood into the larynx and trachea. Prompt recognition of the problem is essential and suction toilet of the pharynx and, if necessary, the trachea and main bronchi can conceivably be required. This latter can be accomplished by passage of a suction catheter down an endotracheal tube passed through the larynx. If this tracheal toilet is performed remember to ensure the proper oxygenation of the patient between suction attempts because it is very easy to produce anoxia by passing a suction catheter into the bronchial tree — in addition to any foreign material, the suction catheter removes gases in considerable quantities and this, of course, includes oxygen.

Nasotracheal tubes can be passed deep to the mucosa of the posterior pharyngeal wall on rare occasions and this can be demonstrated on laryngoscopic examination which will reveal the bulge caused by the tube deep to the pharyngeal mucosa. Should this occur, immediately withdraw the tube and make no further attempts at nasotracheal intubation. Instead, pass an endotracheal tube orally and insert a firm pharyngeal pack. The author has only known of one instance of this complication and that in a personal report by a colleague.

5

Complications and precautions in dental anaesthesia

It is patently obvious to all hospital-based anaesthetists working in dental surgeries remote from the hospital environment, that however well a surgery is equipped it will never be as well endowed with the back-up services as the district hospital with all sorts of medical and ancillary staff on hand to help with emergency situations. In the dental surgery the anaesthetist is virtually alone and he must prepare himself as best he can to cope with emergency situations unsupported. Resuscitatory drugs must be readily accessible where an almost untrained assistant can speedily bring them to his hand. The most certain way of dealing with potential disasters is to avoid these situations when possible. The surest way of doing this is to ensure there is an enquiry into the medical history before an appointment for general anaesthesia is made and in this respect the dental surgeon can be relied upon to obtain such information. In addition, the instruction leaflet given to patients making an appointment for general anaesthesia and the list of questions, detailed later (page 43), based on those used for out-patients at Liverpool Dental School are helpful. In cases of doubt the author finds that the dentist will supply him with enough information to decide whether to communicate with the patient's general practitioner or examine hospital records — a very useful procedure frequently carried out — or pay a visit to the patient at his home after making an appointment to do so. It may well be that information obtained from such sources makes one advise that the dental operation be performed in hospital on an in-patient basis. Whatever decision is reached it must be in the patient's best interests and for no other reason. In an attempt to help others avoid emergency situations in the course of out-patient dental anaesthesia a number of these potential hazards are discussed and guidance is offered concerning how these conditions can be treated and how they may develop.

1. Hypotension
Probably the most serious complication of dental anaesthesia is hypotension during the administration of the anaesthetic. While this

is most likely to happen in the elderly — and a surprising number of elderly patients attend for dental extractions — it does happen at all ages, more often in the highly emotional person. The anaesthetist must be able to see the colour of the patient throughout the administration, watching for pallor especially of sudden onset. The anaesthetist can often manage to apply a finger tip to the facial, temporal or carotid pulses but his other activities— holding firmly the head and nasal mask — may prevent him sensitively feeling a pulse. The moment hypotension is even suspected the back of the dental chair must be lowered to prevent cerebral hypoxia and measures instituted to ensure oxygenation of the lungs. Fainting can occur with some patients, prompted simply by the act of sitting in the dental chair, though this phenomenon is probably a less frequent occurrence than formerly because of better relations between dentist and patient and a consequent reduction of patient fear. Fainting may also occur during the introduction of an intravenous needle or during the injection of the methohexitone in nervous patients and, of course, hypotension may occur due to the central or peripheral effects of the methohexitone or the halothane. Fainting, or hypotensive episodes, may also occur during gaseous induction and maintenance, especially if high concentrations of halothane are used for too long. Whatever the cause and whenever it occurs, hypotension must always be treated by discontinuing the administration of halothane and by the immediate levelling of the back of the chair and raising the legs to seat level or above, care being taken to see that oxygen is not only being delivered to the patient but that it is being taken into his lungs either by spontaneous respiration through a clear airway or by ventilation using manual compression of the reservoir bag. Recovery of the blood pressure in the vast majority of instances will occur spontaneously without recourse to drugs, though in rare instances an intravenous injection of a drug such as Vasoxine (methoxamine) will be beneficial.

It may be that prior to anaesthesia the patient reports that he is known to have an abnormally low blood pressure. In these cases it is wise to check the blood pressure and, if in fact it is low, the patient must be treated with special care. He should be anaesthetised supine, or at least with the chair tilted back more than for other patients, the induction agent should be administered more slowly than usual in minimal dosage and special watch made for hypotensive episodes. It is worth while to check that the pre-induction hypotensive state is not associated with anaemia.

2. Respiratory depression
Transitory apnoea or respiratory depression may occur following induction by an intravenous agent, perhaps given too quickly. The

painful stimulation of an extraction invariably corrects this condition. Depression can readily occur, especially in children, if halothane administration at high concentrations — over 2 per cent vapour — is continued for too long. This can be corrected by discontinuing the halothane and aiding ventilation with manual compression of the reservoir bag until normal ventilatory levels are resumed. Whatever the cause, manual ventilation must be commenced if depression occurs for more than a very short time — probably 15 seconds is the limit. Respiratory depression can also occur in the emphysematous patient who can over breathe due to the surgical stimulus, or even just nervousness, and wash out his normally high alveolar CO_2 levels. The author has had such an experience and consequently views the severely emphysematous patient with some apprehension. Certainly patients with a very severe degree of emphysema should be dealt with in hospital where they can be cared for postoperatively for a much longer period with plenty of medical and ancillary help available.

3. Regurgitation and vomiting
Regurgitation and vomiting may occur during induction or maintenance of anaesthesia but in a long experience has been found to be rare in properly prepared patients. What is more common is vomiting after the administration has ceased and consciousness has been regained. This occurs most often in the highly nervous, apprehensive child who has had a gaseous induction and possibly expects to be sick afterwards because of a previous experience or tales told to him by friends or relations. The apprehension certainly delays the emptying of the stomach and one is often surprised to find that the vomited food was ingested very many hours beforehand. In cases where the child is extremely apprehensive and will tolerate an intravenous injection, this method of induction is often best if one is to retain the confidence of the child — and his parents — for future occasions, should a return visit prove necessary at a later date. The possibility of vomiting and more particularly regurgitation, makes it essential for each surgery room used for general anaesthetics to be equipped with powerful suction apparatus, of the high volume displacement type, for use in clearing the pharynx of regurgitated gastric contents. Naturally, should such regurgitation occur, the chairback is immediately lowered beyond the horizontal so that gravity may aid the removal of foreign material from the vicinity of the larynx and trachea.

4. Tetany
The author has experienced one case of tetany, occurring during the recovery period. This 14-year-old, very apprehensive boy hyperventi-

lated as consciousness was regained. He developed early carpopedal spasm and was beginning to lose consciousness again despite repeated requests to breathe normally instead of panting rapidly as he was doing. The condition was only relieved when he was made to rinse his mouth out repeatedly for several minutes thus breaking the vicious circle by concentrating his attention on rinsing and spitting into the bowl. It is of interest to note that upon questioning the parents it turned out that the patient had had an appendicectomy six months earlier and following this the surgeon had told the parents that there had been some difficulty with his respiration postoperatively. Two junior anaesthetists had attended him at the operation but had noted no difficulties in his case record and could not recall the occasion. Likewise, the ward records did not refer to any difficulty. The surgeon concerned could not recall the incident either but we are left wondering if there had been a similar tetanic incident following his earlier anaesthetic. Certainly on the occasion of the dental anaesthetic the boy developed true tetany which resolved when he resumed a normal respiratory pattern.

5. Delay in recovery

A slight delay in recovery of consciousness can be a complication but is of minor significance. It is more in the category of a nuisance than anything else — nuisance to the patient, to the surgeon and to the anaesthetist. It is usually due to a misjudgement of the anaesthetic requirement, keeping the halothane on longer than necessary or perhaps giving too large a dose of methohexitone for the patient's requirements. The latter is most likely to arise in children and the elderly.

A prolonged delay in recovery, judged by no observable signs of progressive lightening of unconsciousness over a period of a minute or two, is in a different category entirely and must be viewed with a high degree of concern and an early attempt at a diagnosis should be attempted. Immediately one must think of the possibility of a cerebro-vascular accident perhaps resulting from an undetected hypotensive episode and so the patient must be placed in a supine position with his head at or below heart level to ensure that the brain suffers no further deprivation. Check the pulse and, if possible, the blood pressure. If there is no pulse external cardiac massage must be instituted ensuring that pulmonary ventilation is continued either spontaneously or by intermittent positive pressure ventilation after a rapid endotracheal intubation. If respirations have ceased, and the pulse is adequate, oxygen must be administered by manual compression of a reservoir bag using either a face mask or an endotracheal tube. These measures will help to maintain the vital functions until a definite diagnosis of the trouble is reached or recovery takes place.

The anaesthetist must also consider other causes of coma. A known diabetic patient may be suffering from either hypoglycaemia as a consequence of too large an insulin intake in relation to ingested diet — for example a normal insulin dosage followed by the starvation required prior to the anaesthetic. This should respond to glucose by mouth if at all possible, otherwise intravenous glucose will be required urgently. In the absence of a history of diabetes under treatment, hypoglycaemia could rarely be caused by an insulin secreting tumour but the preanaesthetic questioning should have elucidated any suggestion of this sort of disease. Hyperglycaemia might possibly be a cause of unconsciousness in an untreated diabetic but would almost certainly be accompanied by ketosis with its characteristic odour.

There is always the remote possibility of either a cardiovascular or cerebrovascular incident occurring during general anaesthesia in the dental chair just as it is possible at any other time. The author has personal knowledge of two deaths occurring a few minutes before medical or dental attention was due to take place, one occurring in hospital and one occurring in a dental surgery waiting room in another part of the country. However one must not assume coincidence, should an accident occur. Resuscitative attempts must be instituted immediately one suspects that something is amiss and before a catastrophe has occurred.

6. Oxygen supplies

It must be stated, however obvious it may appear, that a careful watch must be kept on oxygen cyclinders. The dental anaesthetist must be aware at all times of the state of these cylinders, both the one in use and the spare ones. Many surgeries are now using piped gases with very large cylinders and so long as the anaesthetist is aware of the state of the cylinders at the start of the session he need only check occasionally on the one in use during the course of the session, provided it started the session in a healthy state. Some surgeries have pressure gauges actually in the surgery used for general anaesthetic cases and these are a great help to the anaesthetist but this is not always possible because of the siting of the cylinders in relation to the surgery, or because gases are piped to several surgeries which are all used for general anaesthetic work. There is no excuse nowadays for using an anaesthetic apparatus without a certain knowledge of the state of the oxygen cylinders on the apparatus. Even if elderly

McKesson Simplor machines are in use, they can, as described later, be converted to carry pressure gauges indicating the contents of the oxygen cylinders.

7. Regularly administered drugs

Advances in medical treatment are continually occurring, new drugs are frequently coming into general use, life expectancy is greater and people continue to lead active lives supported by these drugs in spite of previously life-threatening diseases. These new drugs are often highly potent and can pose problems for the anaesthetist who wishes to administer other potent drugs which may well increase the hazard to the patient. In view of the plethora of new drugs often appearing under different trade names, it is advisable to have an up-to-date copy of the Monthly Index of Medical Specialities (MIMS) in each dental surgery. The chief categories of drugs which we must consider are these:

- a. Sedative or anti-depressive drugs
- b. Anti-hypertensive drugs
- c. Steroids
- d. Drugs given for asthma
- e. Digoxin and other cardiac drugs

a. *Sedative and anti-depressive drugs* are very commonly encountered in the dental surgery sometimes in relatively heavy dosage. These patients have to be dealt with in their normal pharmacological state and so require rather careful handling. Intravenous barbiturates and inhaled halothane have both to be administered with great care. The injection is given more slowly than usual lest the circulatory stabilising mechanism is disturbed and a hypotensive episode is precipitated which will happen more readily than with patients not on these drugs. When possible, MAOI (monoamine oxidase inhibitors) are stopped for two weeks prior to the anaesthetic but it is not always possible to do this. Firstly, the patient, or his general practitioner, may not feel the patient can cope with everyday life without his support from the drug. Secondly, the patient may be in the dental surgery for emergency treatment because of a dental abscess which cannot wait for two weeks. In these circumstances experience has so far shown that these patients may be dealt with safely if carefully handled with a slow intravenous injection of the induction agent and minimal halothane, or preferably no halothane, as for patients taking other sedative drugs.

b. *Anti-hypertensive drugs* should not be interrupted because of an impending general anaesthetic. If these patients require these drugs to keep them free of symptoms of their hypertension and their blood pressures near to normal levels, then they require them more than ever when faced with general anaesthesia. The anaesthetist must expect that their blood pressures are more labile than normotensive patients and should treat them with special care as with the patients on sedative drugs. Extra special watch is kept for hypotensive episodes which must be treated by immediate levelling of the chair and the administration of oxygen.

c. *Previous long-term steroid therapy* requires that the patient be given extra steroids to cover the period of stress. When possible a doubled dose is given at the usual medication time prior to the appointment and hydrocortisone 100 mg is injected intravenously immediately before the methohexitone is given. Increased steroid dosage for several days postoperatively is advisable, gradually reducing to the normal maintenance dose after 4–6 days. When an emergency extraction is being performed and there is no opportunity for an increased dosage prior to the anaesthetic, intravenous hydrocortisone 100 mg is given, as described, before the methohexitone and the postoperative steroid regime described above is instituted.

d. *Drugs taken regularly for asthma* should be continued in normal dosage up to and following the anaesthetic. This advice covers oral drugs as well as the use of inhalants. Unfortunately many patients have a tendency to miss out medication of this sort prior to their visit to the dental surgery just when they are in special need of their maintenance therapy. In practice it is found that these patients can be given a carefully administered anaesthetic without incident but one must be prepared to give intravenous hydrocortisone or bronchodilator drugs should an episode of bronchospasm occur.

e. *Digoxin and other drugs acting on the heart* should be continued uninterrupted before and after anaesthesia, in their normal dosage. Whether or not these patients can be dealt with on an out-patient basis for dental anaesthesia is a separate matter. The dental surgeon elicits information from the patient at an earlier visit regarding his health and where there is any suggestion of doubt he should warn the anaesthetist in advance giving him the patient's name, address and general practitioner's name. Enquiries can then be made through the patient's own doctor and the hospital records, and even by a visit to the patient's home where he may be interviewed and examined. These enquiries can form the basis of the decision concerning whether the patient is suitable to be anaesthetised in the dental chair or whether he should be admitted to hospital for the operative procedure. Major factors in determining fitness for anaesthesia include an assessment of exercise tolerance, the degree of dyspnoea present and the presence of oedema. A decrease of exercise tolerance inconsistent with age, dyspnoea with only moderate exercise or the presence of ankle oedema not due to local factors such as disease of veins should be taken as an indication not to go ahead with general anaesthesia outside of the hospital environment. Again, these patients, if considered fit for out-patient dental anaesthesia must be treated with very great care and especially with a slow intravenous injection of the induction agent. Remember that most of these patients have an increased circulation time and that, therefore, they will take longer to demonstrate the effect of intravenously injected drugs. Before anaesthetising these patients, two or three minutes' preoxygenation with them breathing 100 per cent oxygen is recommended, and is readily accepted by these patients when its object is explained to them.

8. Epilepsy
This disease tends to be disregarded somewhat as a hazard when considering the patient for dental anaesthesia, because a barbiturate is being administered intravenously and this one would expect to damp down cerebral activity. However the author has had an experience which has caused him to be more wary of this disease. A young man of 21 years of age, an epileptic of many years' standing on regular medication with phenytoin, was presented for anaesthesia. He admitted to having a seizure about every 2 or 3 months. He was given methohexitone, nitrous oxide and oxygen for the removal of 3 teeth and this was uneventful. Almost 10 minutes after the conclusion of the anaesthesia, having rinsed his mouth and spoken rationally, he began to jactitate and lost consciousness. It was a further 30 minutes before he was sufficiently recovered to be taken home by his father. It now came to light that his fits occurred at home mostly when he was awakening from sleep. Some months later his dentist advised further multiple extractions. This time the procedure was carried out in hospital with premedication followed by endotracheal anaesthesia and was uneventful.

9. Sickle cell disease
The chances of encountering sickle cell disease or the trait has increased in recent years with the increase in the immigrant population and this affects some districts of Britain more than others. The advice an anaesthetist can obtain from the literature varies, sometimes varying with the interest of the writer of the book or article

for it is found that some physicians show an outdated understanding of anaesthesia, still suggesting that hypoxia plays some role in dental anaesthesia. Whatever the viewpoint, however, it would seem wise not to anaesthetise patients with sickle cell disease outside of hospital. Those with the trait are in a different category and it would seem wise to establish the relative proportions of HbS and HbA. If the proportion of HbS were low, say 25 per cent or less, and the dental operation were of a minor character — for example, one or two teeth for extraction — the writer would be prepared to anaesthetise them in the dental surgery. In patients with only 25 per cent HbS, according to Lehmann and Huntsman in 'Man's Haemoglobins', sickling does not begin until the PO_2 is less than 25 mmHg. The difficulty arises in being able to have electrophoretic tests carried out prior to surgery in order to establish the relative proportions of HbS and HbA. The real deciding factors seem to be whether the case can be managed without the risk of hypoxia — which very rarely occurs in the well managed anaesthetic in any case — and whether or not the case can be better managed in hospital anyway. Any patient who has origins in the West Indies or Africa ought to be referred to the haematology department of the local hospital or have a specimen of blood sent to them for testing. There is available a pack which can be used in the surgery for carrying out this test but it has a limited shelf life and its use by the occasional 'amateur' technician does not give reliable results. Use of the laboratory facilities of the local hospital is much more reliable.

10. Pregnancy

It is established that on occasions halothane administered during pregnancy is a cause of miscarriage and premature labour. It is consequently unwise to administer halothane to pregnant patients. As the manufacturers of methohexitone, in their descriptive leaflet which accompanies each bottle of 'Brietal', warn users that the drug's effect in pregnancy is not established, the dental anaesthetist is left in a quandary. The author's practice has been to use methohexitone for induction and to maintain anaesthesia with nitrous oxide and oxygen alone though on rare occasions it has proved necessary in the interests of smooth anaesthesia to add a little halothane vapour. Over a considerable number of years this practice has not caused any difficulty from the point of view of premature labour.

Another difficulty associated with late pregnancy is the splinting of the diaphragm by the sheer mass of the pregnant uterus. It is felt that these patients are best dealt with in a slightly more upright posture than for other dental procedures simply to allow free diaphragmatic movement. In both early and late pregnancy prolonged anaesthesia for dental clearances is not encouraged, anaesthesia in the main being confined to short anaesthetics for a few extractions, mostly of an emergency nature. If, however, there is any previous history of miscarriages or premature labour, general anaesthesia is avoided if possible.

If any of the chairside assistants who normally help during general anaesthetic sessions is pregnant she should be advised not to undertake these duties where she may be subjected to an atmosphere containing halothane vapour. This applies even when some means of scavenging the halothane vapour is in use.

11. Angina and ischaemic heart disease

Patients suffering from these complaints should be viewed in the high risk category. Al-Khishali *et al*. found in a series of healthy patients a high incidence of abnormal cardiac rhythms and of tachycardia, leading them to conclude that 'the presence of tachycardia and arrhythmia in patients with ischaemic heart disease is a potentially dangerous situation'. With this the author heartily concurs but would add a warning that those patients whose angina is obviously deteriorating with the passage of time are also in a very high risk category. In short, only those patients whose angina is mild and stable and who have no tachycardia or arrhythmia should be considered for out-patient general anaesthesia. All others should definitely be referred for hospital in-patient treatment.

If it is decided that a patient with ischaemic heart disease can be safely dealt with in the dental surgery he must be anaesthetised with great care. The patient should be semi–reclining as usual and before any attempt is made to anaesthetise him he should have two or three minutes of pre-oxygenation, breathing 100 per cent oxygen. Thereafter, a slow intravenous injection of methohexitone may be given while carefully watching his pulse, colour and respiration. Remember his circulation time is probably increased. Should there be any deterioration whatsoever revealed by these observations, the patient must be lowered immediately to a horizontal position, the injection having been discontinued, and resuscitative measures instituted as indicated.

The best advice in selecting these patients for general anaesthesia in the dental surgery is — if in doubt about the fitness, DON'T.

12. Acute respiratory disease

A common problem for the dental anaesthetist is the patient with a cold or recovering from one. If the infection is severe the patient is unlikely to attend the surgery at all invariably telephoning to say he is too unwell to attend. The minor respiratory problem mostly consists of the patient with a 'blocked nose'. If the nasal passages can be cleared by blowing, the anaesthetic may be administered with care but if the nasal passages cannot be cleared to give a free flow of air during normal respirations the operative procedure is better delayed for at least a week until the patient has recovered.

13. Allergic skin reaction

An 18 year old girl was given methohexitone 75 mg intravenously and anaesthesia was maintained with only nitrous oxide and oxygen delivered by a Quantiflex R.A. machine for the extraction of two teeth. Ten minutes later the patient complained of a mild urticarial rash over her face, neck and body. After thirty minutes this had worsened and she was taken to the Casualty Department of the local hospital where she was given an injection of Piriton (chlor-pheniramine) 10 mg which rapidly produced relief. A supply of tablets was given to be taken for the next few days. There was no recurrence or further complication. It is interesting to note that two years previously this patient was given a similar anaesthetic for an extraction. On her way home she developed a mild irritant rash of her neck and chest which did not persist. In fact she thought so little of it that she did not mention it until after the second more severe episode occurred. She had no other experience of taking barbiturates. It would seem wise that on a possible future occasion a non-barbiturate intravenous agent be used for induction or perhaps even a gaseous induction.

14. Diabetic Patients

Diabetic patients pose a difficult problem to the dental anaesthetist. For practical purposes the author divides them into three categories:

a. *Diabetic patients controlled by diet alone*
These patients may be dealt with in the normal manner, with the usual restriction of food or drink for at least four hours pre-operatively. Patients in this group and in section (b) below who may have difficulty in managing a normal diet post-operatively because they have had so many teeth extracted, should be guided regarding liquid diet equivalents.

b. *Diabetic patients well controlled by drug therapy who are having only a few teeth extracted*
If these patients can, with certainty, control their diabetic state by the intelligent variation of their dietary intake and drug therapy with advice from the anaesthetist, can also be operated upon first thing in the morning so that they may more easily judge their diet and the drug

D

dosage to match it and are for the extraction of only a very few teeth so that their ability to eat and drink afterwards is not impaired, then the author is prepared to anaesthetise them. If even one of these conditions cannot be met with certainty then they must be referred for hospital in-patient extractions where there is plenty of medical and nursing aid to deal with any crisis. If the patient is not being treated with insulin but by tablets a word of warning is relevant. If the tablets are of the sulphonylurea group such as Chloropropamide or Tolbutamide then the above advice is relevant. If, however, the tablets are of the biguanide type, Phenformin or Metformin, it is advisable for them to be treated in hospital because they are prone to lactic acidosis, a potentially fatal condition.

If all the above conditions have been met and a decision has been reached to anaesthetise the patient in the dental surgery, then the patient arrives at the surgery for, say, 9 a.m. having had nothing whatsoever by mouth that morning and no drugs. The anaesthesia is administered in the normal manner and the patient is allowed home with instructions to resume his dietary and drug regime for the day, starting of course, an hour or so later than normal. Patients who have had extractions because of infection, may require the dose of oral diabetic agents to be reduced after the operation and subsidence of the infection.

c. *Diabetic patients on insulin or ones who are badly controlled by any means, who are having many teeth extracted.*
These patients should be operated upon in hospital where a full medical team can supervise the pre-operative and post-operative management.

Really, if there is any doubt at all about the management of any diabetic patient he should be taken into hospital. Even with patients in either of the first two categories who, it is suggested, may be treated as out-patients, much depends upon the experience of the anaesthetist with diabetic patients.

15. Other contra-indications to out-patient dental anaesthesia
It would be wise not to anaesthetise on an out-patient basis any patient suffering from oedema of the floor of the mouth and acute swellings of the neck such as Ludwig's angina and quinsy. These should be hospitalized. So too should patients suffering from thyrotoxicosis, haemophilia and severe degrees of anaemia as well as those mentioned above suffering from severe cardiac and pulmonary disease and the diabetic patients described above. There is of course an absolute contra-indication to the use of barbiturates in patients with porphyria so intravenous methohexitone must not be used for induction of anaesthesia.

16. Routine instructions to patients

The preparation of the patient for general anaesthesia for dental surgery begins with the weeding out of the unsuitable patient and the establishing in the anaesthetist's mind of relevant factors in the patient's health and history. The author finds it useful to himself and his dental colleagues for them to present to the patient at the time his appointment is made, a questionnaire card (see below) based on one used in the Liverpool Dental School and illustrated by Dr Gough Hughes in General Anaesthesia (ed. Grey, T. C. and Nunn, T. F., published by Butterworth, S.: London, Boston).

PATIENTS FOR GENERAL ANAESTHESIA

Have you suffered from any of the following conditions, now or in the past?

1. Heart disease
2. Lung disease including a persistent cough
3. Rheumatic Fever
4. High or low blood pressure
5. Kidney disease
6. Diabetes, hyperthyroidism, porphyria
7. Blood disease, anaemia, excessive bleeding tendencies
8. Epilepsy, fainting attacks
9. Nervous trouble

Are you
a) Allergic to anything?
b) On any medicine or drugs?
c) Pregnant?

Having obtained a satisfactory history and made an appointment for general anaesthesia, instructions are best given in two forms, verbally and in writing. Verbal instructions are given not to have anything to eat or drink for four hours prior to the appointment, to come to the surgery with a responsible adult who will accompany the patient home, not to drive a car or operate machinery after the anaesthetic until the next day, and so on. These instructions are reinforced by written instructions handed to the patient at the time the appointment is made and which he is asked to read carefully. A copy of the instructions issued by the author is illustrated (see below). One of the more important points which requires emphasis is that which instructs the patient to be accompanied *to the surgery* by a responsible adult. Without this specific instruction patients are liable to leave their escort outside in a car some distance away or else to send him or her off on a shopping expedition. The escort must come into the surgery premises with the patient and wait until he is ready to be escorted home.

Any personal illness, including coughs and colds, should be reported to the dental surgeon. If you are taking any tablets or other medicine prescribed by your doctor, please find out from him the correct name of the drug and report this to your dentist some days prior to the date of the anaesthetic.

NO FOOD OR DRINK SHOULD HAVE BEEN TAKEN FOR AT LEAST 4 HOURS BEFORE THE APPOINTMENT AND THE LAST MEAL SHOULD BE LIGHT AND EASILY DIGESTIBLE.

All patients must be accompanied *to the surgery* by an adult.

Any tight clothing should be loosened. Bowels and bladder should be empty. Patients, particularly children, should visit the toilet before attending the surgery.

Patients must not drive any vehicle or operate any machinery until the following day.

Afterwards, do not use mouth washes vigorously.

NAME _____

DATE AND TIME OF APPOINTMENT _____

6

Apparatus

It is proposed to discuss briefly three groups of dental anaesthetic machines, the ones the author finds most commonly in use for dental anaesthesia. These are the Quantiflex models manufactured and sold by Cyprane, the various McKesson models, and the Boyle apparatus.

Quantiflex apparatus
There are two models, the 'R.A.' machine designed, according to Cyprane, for relative analgesia, and the 'M.D.M.' model — the Dental Monitored Dial Mixer.

The Quantiflex R.A. Mark II
This machine is considered to be the most suitable apparatus available at present for dental anaesthesia because, firstly, it is convenient to use but, equally important, it has many safety features. The convenience arises from the fact that, once the anaesthetist has pre-set his gas flows, the gases are then controlled by a single on-off switch. This has the important advantage that there is no time spent twiddling control knobs to increase gas flows; immediately the switch is raised the gases flow at the pre-determined rates, both the oxygen and nitrous oxide being controlled by this one switch. Nothing is more frustrating during a busy anaesthetic session than having to turn on two separate flowmeters, as in the Boyle type apparatus, for this would occupy one hand for valuable seconds at the beginning — and, even more importantly, at the end of the anaesthetic when there are more urgent things to be done while attending to the patient. Remembering, of course, that the care of the patient takes first priority, the prompt cessation of gas flows at the earliest opportunity conserves gases, reduces the pollution of the atmosphere in the surgery and reduces costs, as either the anaesthetist or the dentist is paying for these gases.

The most important features of this machine, however, are its many safety factors. First of all it will not deliver less than 3 litres of oxygen per minute. The nitrous oxide will not flow unless the oxygen is also

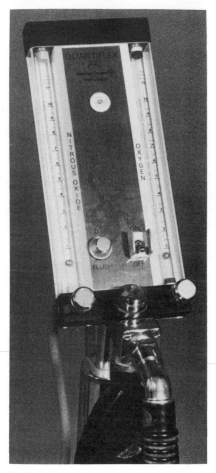

Fig. 6.1 Quantiflex R.A. Apparatus

running. There is an automatic cut off of the nitrous oxide flow if there is any failure of the oxygen supply. With the nitrous oxide flow rate at its maximum of 10 litres per minute the minimum oxygen content of the mixture is 23 per cent which can be exceeded by increasing the oxygen flow above the minimum 3 litres per minute or by decreasing the flow of nitrous oxide. There is, of course, an oxygen flush valve operated independently of the on-off switch by a button which may be depressed but not locked on. Depression of this button gives a rapid supply of 100 per cent oxygen. It should be noted that in this apparatus, as well as in many other dental anaesthetic machines, the oxygen flush valve is situated proximal to the vaporiser which makes it absolutely imperative that the vaporiser is turned off before the emergency oxygen button is used. There is a guard around the on-off switch designed to prevent accidental operation of the switch but in practice it is found that the switch is not vulnerable to accidental operation. There is, also, a non-return valve behind a fresh gas outlet which prevents the possibility of the patient re-breathing to and from the reservoir bag. If the fail safe systems, which ensure that nitrous oxide does not flow without oxygen, should really break down, there is an air intake valve which introduces room air into the system. All these features combine to ensure more than adequate oxygenation at all times, provided of course the patient's respirations are free and unobstructed.

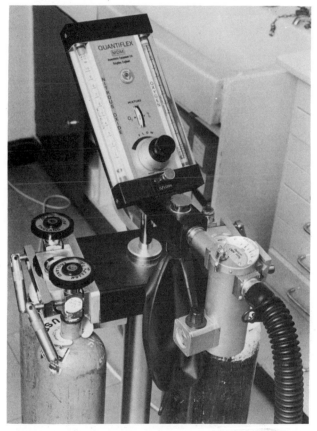

Fig. 6.2 Quantiflex M.D.M. Apparatus with Penlon OMV 50 Vaporiser

The Quantiflex Dental Monitored Dial Mixer (Dental M.D.M.)
This apparatus (see Heath *et al.*, 1973) is very similar to the Quantiflex R.A. machine. The oxygen percentage is determined by a mixer control with a minimum oxygen content of 30 per cent and graduated

from 30 per cent to 100 per cent oxygen. The flow is regulated by a knob which is turned in an anti-clockwise direction to increase the gas flows which are demonstrated by the clearly demarcated flowmeters. This allows for lower total gas flows than the R.A. apparatus. The author finds it convenient to use a total gas flow of 10 litres per minute with 30 per cent oxygen — that is, 3 litres of oxygen and 7 litres of nitrous oxide — during both gaseous induction and the maintenance of anaesthesia. His only criticisms of this apparatus are these — it is less convenient and slightly more time consuming to have to turn the flow knob and secondly, an oxygen content of 30 per cent leads to a slightly longer gaseous induction time than the R.A. machine when it is delivering 23–25 per cent oxygen. Both machines have clearly laid out faces, conveniently set at an angle of 45° for easy reading of the settings.

McKesson anaesthetic apparatus

Probably the most commonly found apparatus and the most popular among dental anaesthetists during the last twenty years or more has been the McKesson Simplor machine. This had certain disadvantages — one obvious and others which were not generally appreciated. The

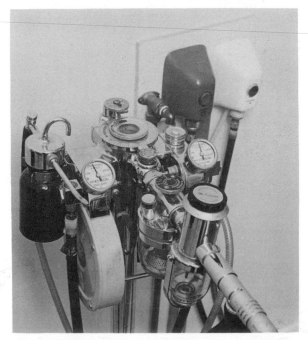

Fig. 6.3 McKesson Simplor machine with a McKesson Trilene vaporiser and a Goldman halothane vaporiser in series

earlier Simplor apparatus was supplied with gases from cylinders located on the stand with no means of knowing how much oxygen or nitrous oxide was contained in these cylinders. There was only an indication that the gases were reaching the apparatus and these indicating dials, rapidly and without much warning, dropped to zero when the cylinders emptied. When the apparatus is connected to piped gases, the state of the centrally located large cylinders can readily be checked before and during an anaesthetic session. For this important reason the author felt it essential that the McKesson Simplor unit was connected to piped gases. However the situation has changed recently. The McKesson Company now have available conversion units for these early models and, by fitting two reducing valves, two high pressure gauges and four non-return valves, it is now possible to be aware of the amount of gases, particularly oxygen, contained in each cylinder. The cost of this conversion, early in 1979, is about £128.

The new model of the Simplor apparatus has a safety cut out valve which operates if the oxygen supply fails. If this should occur the patient will breath air through this safety valve. However, it is still possible, with the new model as well as with the earlier ones, for the apparatus to be set to deliver 100 per cent nitrous oxide and there is still a temptation among a few anaesthetists to use low oxygen concentrations during induction as was common practice many years ago. Low oxygen concentrations at any time are to be deprecated and are quite indefensible. When using this type of machine the author pre-sets the oxygen concentration at 25 per cent and generally leaves this control strictly undisturbed except when he wishes for some special reason to raise the oxygen level. The gas flow is conveniently controlled by a single control marked 'Pressure', which increases the gas flow as it is turned in a clockwise direction. It is possible, by reducing the amount of 'pressure' used, to deliver gases only intermittently during the patient's inspiration. This 'demand flow' was a recognised technique many years ago but roundly condemned by, among others, Courville (1936), Goldman (1958), Nainby-Luxmoore (1967) and Allen et al. (1969). The author has been told that the 'demand flow' technique is becoming popular again in some anaesthetic practices. This technique has the advantage of possibly conserving gases and, if so, would be less expensive to administer but it is firmly believed that free flowing gases are safer, give a much smoother anaesthetic and pick up halothane vapour more consistently.

Doubts have been expressed in recent years about the performance of the McKesson apparatus. If the free flow of gases is obstructed, oxygen concentrations can be unpredictable (Nainby-Luxmoore, 1967). In practice, however, it does not matter to the patient what gases are being delivered to him if respiratory obstruction has occurred until, of course, he takes his first unobstructed breath. What is of paramount importance is to clear the obstructed airway whatever the cause, and to ensure that, once the respiration is free, the gases being delivered contain at least 25 per cent oxygen. Although the early Simplor machines do not come up to the British Safety Standards they continue to be used widely. It is strongly recommended that they be used with piped gases or have the conversion units, described earlier, fitted to them. The author believes that these machines, with the piped gases or the conversion unit, provided they are carefully used in the manner described, with the anaesthetist being aware of their limitations, and, very important, are serviced regularly, are satisfactory machines for dental anaesthesia. The newer models with their safety cut out in the event of oxygen failure are, of course, much to be preferred.

The McKesson Equipment Company, now of Chesterfield, have introduced several RA/GA models suitable for either relative analgesia or general anaesthesia. The earlier models are called the '7 series' and the latest one is called the Consul 881 RA/GA. These are continuous flow machines. Gas flows for general anaesthesia are controlled by two flowmeters in their '7' series models. By turning a switch on the side of the apparatus to the RA position, the minimum oxygen flow rate becomes three litres per minute. Should the oxygen supply fail the nitrous oxide is automatically cut off and a special air valve comes into operation allowing the patient to breath air only. McKesson's newest model, the Consul 881 RA/GA, gives an oxygen percentage reading and has a simple control knob to adjust the flow. There is a visual warning red light should the oxygen line pressure fall below 60 p.s.i; when the pressure is maintained at 60 p.s.i. a green light is shown. This type of apparatus obviously has none of the faults of the early Simplor machines where oxygen concentrations can be upset in the presence of an obstruction to the flow of gases.

Boyle apparatus

While any of the available Boyle machines are perfectly capable of delivering oxygen and nitrous oxide at whatever flow rates the anaesthetist wishes and can be relied upon to do so provided the gas cylinders are functioning, they are not considered by the author to be ideally suited for dental anaesthesia. There is the inconvenience of turning on and off two separate flowmeters which is, as mentioned before, unnecessarily laborious and distracting from the anaesthetist's prime concern, the patient. Further, these machines are usually of a height which allows a seated anaesthetist in theatre to see the level of the bobbins conveniently — but the dental anaesthetist is standing, and consequently his eyes are at too high a level to read conveniently the gas flows in the vertical flowmeters. This problem is satisfactorily overcome in the Quantiflex machines by inclining the flowmeter head at 45° to the vertical so that the small balls registering the gas flows can be readily seen.

Halothane vaporisers
The vaporiser must satisfy two criteria. Firstly it must not be too heavy as the dental anaesthetist will be expected to carry it with him in his equipment bag. Secondly it must be able to deliver enough halothane to provide anaesthesia and to do so within safe limits and, if possible, in a known vapour concentration. There seem to the author to be two ways of accomplishing this, depending upon how much money the anaesthetist is prepared to invest, but the cost differences are only marginal.

a. *Penlon OMV fifty vaporiser*

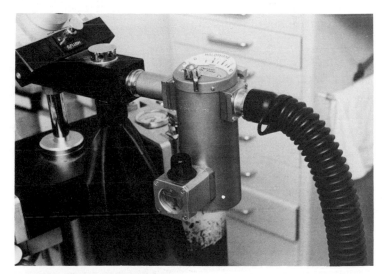

Fig. 6.4 The Penlon OMV 50 Vaporiser

This vaporiser weighs 1.4 kg, holds 50 ml of halothane and is calibrated from 0 to 4.0 per cent of halothane with calibrations denoting each 0.5 per cent of vapour. A sight glass reveals the halothane contained within, so that the anaesthetist should know when the vaporiser is nearly empty. It is temperature buffered rather than fully temperature compensated so that with continuous flow over a period there will be a slight temperature drop and with this a small reduction in the vapour concentrations below the value of the settings on the dial — a fail-safe mechanism of sorts. The manufacturers claim in their literature that a setting of 2 per cent, while at 22°C, will deliver the set concentration but a reduction in the temperature to, for example, 16°C will reduce the concentration to 1.8 per cent vapour, for the same dial setting. Higher settings produce a slightly greater drop in concentration with similar temperature falls. Lower settings, on the other hand, retain their accuracy with the same temperature changes. High flow rates produce a vapour concentration lower than that indicated by the setting when at the higher levels (a setting of 3 per cent at 10 litres per minute delivers 2.2 per cent halothane vapour while a 2 per cent setting at the same flow rate delivers about 1.7 per cent halothane) but the concentration remains fairly constant even with high flow rates when the setting is at 1 per cent. Even with these moderate inconsistencies in vapour concentrations with increased flow rates and reductions in temperature, this OMV Fifty Vaporiser is a good, small halothane vaporiser available for dental anaesthesia today provided the weight does not prove an inconvenience and the price of about £146 can be faced.

b. *Cyprane Drawover Fluotec Vaporiser*

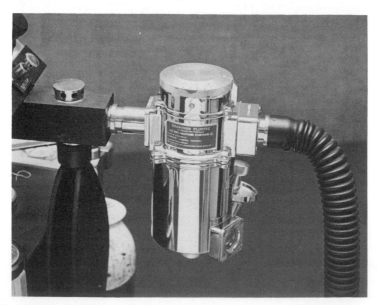

Fig. 6.5 Cyprane Drawover Fluotec Vaporiser

This vaporiser weighs 2.35 kg and is much heavier than the Penlon model. However it is temperature compensated rather than temperature buffered and, for gas flow rates between 6 and 16 litres per minute, delivers fairly accurately the percentage vapour for which the vaporiser is set — it is more accurate than the Penlon. It holds 85 ml of halothane as against the 50 ml of the Penlon model and is calibrated up to 5 per cent in increments of 0.5 per cent. It is a highly efficient vaporiser for dental anaesthesia and its only point of criticism when compared to the Penlon vaporiser is its considerable weight. If this is not an important factor, it will be found to be more efficient in terms of vapour concentration than the Penlon. Although the vaporiser carries a label stating that it is designed for use with a patient demand anaesthetic machine and not for use in closed or semi-closed anaesthetic circuits it works well with continuous flow machines such as the Quantiflex apparatus made by the same manufacturer.

This vaporiser costs slightly less than the Penlon model and currently sells at about £135.

c. *The Goldman Vaporiser*

In practice, the author has found the simple Goldman Vaporiser — which has been on the market much longer than the two previously described models — to be almost equally useful and less costly, but it is only less costly if he uses a single Goldman Vaporiser. The author believes that it delivers inadequate levels of halothane vapour and recommends the use of two vaporisers in series. The cost of two Goldman Vaporisers is at present £136.30.

The Goldman Vaporiser does not have markings to indicate vapour concentrations, only marks indicating how far round the control knob has been moved. Experience with the Goldman will soon reveal to the anaesthetist the settings required to produce the desired effect. Each Goldman Vaporiser will be found to be slightly different from others and the anaesthetist will learn to appreciate which deliver slightly more halothane than others. When purchased, the Goldman will have a leaflet indicating the maximum halothane delivered by designated gas flows. However, no attempt is made with this apparatus to buffer temperature changes. Consequently the anaesthetist will discover that, in use, the temperature will rapidly fall and lead to a rapid reduction in the vapour concentration being delivered. Although this reduction does take place, it rarely if ever proves an inconvenience and in fact ensures that high vapour concentration cannot be delivered to the patient for more than a minute or two. In an attempt to overcome the possibility of lower than desirable vapour concentrations during induction, the author for many years used two Goldman Vaporisers in series. Both were used during a gaseous induction one usually being shut off as maintenance began. If the operation is known to be of a very brief duration, such as the extraction of one or perhaps even two deciduous teeth, both vaporisers can usually be switched off immediately prior to the extractions. In practice, using two Goldman Vaporisers in series the author has found that each individual vaporiser will deliver up to 2 per cent halothane. There happen to be four designated positions of the on-off switch and in each vaporiser there is little difference in vapour concentrations between the third setting and the fourth, which is fully on. When the two vaporisers are used in series they will at first deliver together up to 3 per cent halothane. However, in a short time — one minute or so — the concentration will fall to 1.7 per cent. This fail-safe mechanism is useful from the safety angle and has not proved a problem in maintenance of anaesthesia. Should anyone wish to avoid the problem of the fairly rapid fall in halothane concentration with the two Goldman Vaporisers in series, the only way to do this is to invest in a Penlon temperature buffered vaporiser, or better still, the Cyprane temperature compensated one.

Expiratory valves
Atmospheric pollution by anaesthetic gases and, particularly halothane vapour is a current problem and can be dealt with in the dental surgery by two simple methods. If the amount of general anaesthetic work in a surgery is considerable it is possible to install expensive and complicated extraction systems but in the author's view this should not be necessary if the anaesthetic sessions are only amounting to one or two hours a week, as is usual.

The most efficient method of dealing with expired halothane vapour is to use the special expiratory valve designed and sold by H. G. East & Co. Ltd. (Sandy Lane West, Littlemore, Oxford), and described by A. P. Adams and others in the *British Dental Journal* (July 20, 1976). This valve allows expired gases, with the halothane vapour, to be channelled by way of lightweight corrugated tubing to a charcoal scavenging cylinder such as the Aldasorber. This system efficiently removes halothane vapour before it can pollute the surgery room and it is quite noticeable that the dentist and his assistants appreciate the absence of the vapour — as soon as the scavenging system is introduced they immediately remark on the fact that they feel more wide awake during the rest of the day and have no headaches at work.

An alternative to the East Valve, used by the author since October 1973 before the introduction of alternatives, is to fasten with thread a

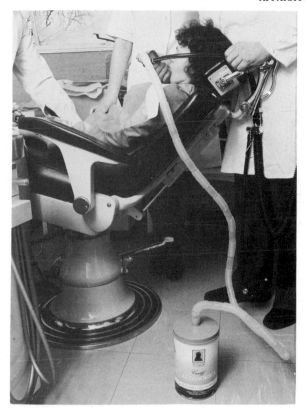

Fig. 6.6 The Cardiff Aldasorber in use with the East Scavenging valve (see also Fig. 2.1)

length of Paul's colostomy tubing over the usual Heidbrink expiratory valve. This tubing leads the expired gases down towards the floor where they are disseminated. Although the halothane vapour is not removed from the atmosphere by charcoal as with the Aldasorber and the East Valve, this system does effectively improve the atmosphere in the anaesthetic room and is greatly appreciated by all those working in the surgery in the same way as the East Valve system is appreciated. This means of improving the working atmosphere was described by the author in the *British Dental Journal* in the issue of 16th July, 1974.

Oronasal masks

The author prefers to use the oronasal masks supplied by the British Oxygen Company for dental anaesthetics. The oral mask has an inflatable cushion enabling the anaesthetist to obtain a gas-tight fit

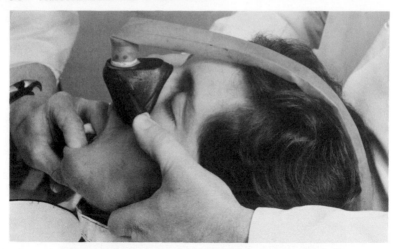

Fig. 6.7 Paul's tubing has been fastened with thread over the Heidbrink valve which is kept fully open because there is a slight back pressure effect of the tubing. Expired gases are carried almost to floor level and away from those working around the patient's head. The use of this tubing was described by the author in the *British Dental Journal* (1974) **132** (2), 44)

over the patient's mouth should he require to use it because of persistant mouth breathing. The ideal combination is the BOC-type oronasal unit with the East scavenging valve.

7

Relative analgesia for conservative dentistry

Up until now we have been concerned only with anaesthesia for extractions and surgical operations. What can be done to relieve the discomfort of conservation work? Immediately we think of local anaesthesia which is tolerated by the great majority of patients. What do we do about the minority though, those who are so apprehensive and nervous that they will not allow the dentist to inject local anaesthetics in their mouths? At the present state of our knowledge, the answer must lie in some form of 'Relative Analgesia'. The term 'Relative Analgesia' was coined by Dr Henry Langa in the United States and refers to a state which can be produced in which painful stimuli are obtunded though the patient may still be aware that manoeuvres are being carried out within the mouth; that is, total senselessness does not occur. In this state the patient can still be co-operative. Above all other considerations, however, the patient's health and survival must not be placed at risk. Here then is where the arguments begin over what is a safe method of producing 'Relative Analgesia'.

To begin with, what is not safe? In recent years it was a fairly common practice for dentists to use intermittent methohexitone given as an initial dose followed by intermittent small supplementary doses given as seemed necessary using as the indication, patient movement and other signs of lightening of the anaesthesia. Respiration is spontaneous and it is usual for the patient to breathe room air through his nose. Problems arise when either apnoea occurs because of too large a dose of methohexitone or when respiratory obstruction occurs. The advocates of this technique used to deny that either of these circumstances regularly occurred but an important paper by Professor Robinson and his colleagues (Wise *et al.*, 1969) showed that both circumstances did in fact occur only too frequently and they could occur without the operator being aware of what had happened. This paper, probably aided by a legal action which followed soon afterwards, has led to the techniques of intermittent methohexitone being discredited. In the past large doses of methohexitone could be

E

given over a period, which on the proponents' admission could last for several hours, and the author has seen reports of 400 mg or more being given in these prolonged administrations. However quickly the body disposes of small single doses of methohexitone, these large doses must have resulted in a very prolonged recovery period. Furthermore the advocates of this technique did not regard their treatment as 'general anaesthesia' and not all of them ensured that their patients were properly prepared prior to induction or left the surgery premises accompanied by a responsible adult who would drive them home. One patient drove to the surgery to receive treatment under intermittent methohexitone, had two pints of beer on the way to the surgery and was later allowed to drive himself home unaccompanied.

The current popular method of treating the apprehensive patient is to use intravenous injections of diazepam. The author believes this technique to suffer from many of the drawbacks of methohexitone. The recovery period after an injection of diazepam is long and one would expect most patients to require — even if they are not always allowed it — a prolonged recovery period in the surgery premises before being accompanied home. Here again there is a grave danger of respiratory depression occurring. The author has knowledge of a case described by the dentist as 'respiratory arrest' though perhaps 'severe respiratory depression' might be a more accurate description. The patient required to have artificial respiration using oxygen from an anaesthetic apparatus before recovery occurred. Incidentally, this technique should never be embarked upon without some means of administering oxygen under controlled conditions being immediately available, and the cylinders of oxygen turned on, ready for use. There are problems too with the actual injection of the diazepam. First it has to be injected much more slowly than methohexitone as its effect is more difficult to judge. The sedation occurs more gradually than with methohexitone. Secondly, the preparation is oily and has therefore to be given through a fairly large needle which is more difficult for the less experienced venepuncturist to insert. Thirdly a common complication of the intravenous injection of diazepam is thrombophlebitis. The patient who suffers for several weeks with thrombophlebitis following his injection is not appreciative of the procedure even though he has had amnesia for the event of the conservation treatment. He would be even less appreciative if he knew also that he had been placed in danger of respiratory arrest or obstruction as a result of the attempt to relieve his anxiety.

What means of 'Relative Analgesia' is therefore safe and effective? The author has no doubt whatsoever that the technique recommended by Dr Langa (1976) is the method of choice. It is safe in that there is no danger of deep anaesthesia being produced by mistake, more than adequate oxygenation is ensured, hypotension and respiratory depression are extremely unlikely to be caused by the technique, co-operation is ensured and recovery is completed rapidly.

The apparatus required is of the sort recommended for general anaesthesia, either the Quantiflex R.A. apparatus or the Quantiflex M.D.M. apparatus, or the McKesson RA/GA machine. Dr Langa himself lists twelve suitable machines, including the ones mentioned above, which are available mainly in the United States. The very large number of these machines available for 'Relative Analgesia' in the United States points to its obvious popularity there which is, in the author's view, a good indication of its acceptability by patients.

Dr. Langa in his book stresses the psychological approach to the patient and recommends a lengthy discussion with the patient to explain the procedure. He even recommends that the dentist and his chairside assistants should try out the technique of inhaling the gases themselves in order that they may be able to relate their own experience to their informative talk to the patients. Dr. Langa does point out that patients of long standing in the dental practice who have a relationship of confidence in their dentist's ability to treat them humanely, will be those who will most readily accept the technique. However, it does appear to this author that these patients will also readily accept local anaesthesia for their conservative work. It is the intractable patients who will benefit most from relative analgesia and these will be the most difficult to persuade of the benefits. Time spent in explaining the procedure and its benefits will not be wasted.

First of all one must stress the absence of after effects and the quick recovery. The patient is told that he will feel relaxed and his nervousness and tension will be eliminated. There is a warm, safe feeling, similar to that of mild but pleasant intoxication — without the after effects. If the dentist should decide to supplement the analgesia with a local anaesthetic injection the injection itself will be painless. The patient is told that as the administration of the gases commences he will feel a warm glow passing through his body. There will be a tingling sensation in his extremeties — toes and fingers particularly, and perhaps even of his lips. When talking to the patient of his sensations, stress at all times must be laid on the pleasantness of the experience. Emphasis can be made of the safety of the procedure. The procedure is not, after all, new as nitrous oxide and oxygen have been in use for over a hundred years. The patient must be told that throughout the operation he must breathe entirely through his nose while his mouth is open. Mouth breathing would completely eradicate the analgesic effect.

The chairside assistants must be instructed that during the administration of relative analgesia there must be no noise or conversation. Handling of instruments must be done carefully and quietly. Conversation must be eliminated all together but if speech is absolutely essential it must be conducted in a whisper. The patient's sense of hearing is the one most likely to be disturbed if accidentally or unnecessarily stimulated.

Prior to any decision being made about undertaking dental treatment under the influence of relative analgesia the medical history must be taken. If there is any contra indication to general anaesthesia, relative analgesia must be avoided. The author would also exclude patients suffering from acute upper respiratory tract infections until resolved, anaemia, chronic bronchitis and emphysema, asthma unless very mild, coronary artery disease and patients suffering from orthopnoea from any cause. If there is any doubt whatsoever about the fitness of the patient further enquiries from medical attendants should be made and, if necessary, any indicated investigations completed. As this must be a safe procedure conducted for a situation which is not threatening to life, no patients about whom doubt exists as to their fitness, should be submitted to relative analgesia— or for that matter, general anaesthesia. It may well be that patients who are pregnant or suffer readily from travel sickness are unsuitable candidates.

How then should the administration be conducted? Dr Langa recommends that at the initial visit when the decision to use 'Relative Analgesia' is made, a trial of the method should be undertaken. The Quantiflex MDM apparatus is one of the best machines for the administration of the 'Relative Analgesia'. Its use is described below. The technique should be adapted appropriately when other machines are available.

A special lightweight nasal mask is placed over the patient's nose while 100 per cent oxygen is flowing and the patient is lying supine on the dental chair. The mask should make fairly firm contact with the patient so that there is no leak of gases except through the expiratory valve. This is sometimes difficult if the patient has a bushy moustache. Should the patient experience discomfort due to difficulty in breathing with the mask in place, an air entrainment valve should be half opened and left so until the patient tolerates and accepts the gases. After a minute or two of breathing oxygen, 10 per cent nitrous oxide is introduced and at intervals of one minute this is increased to 20 per cent, 30 per cent and 40 per cent. Finally, two further increments of 5 per cent are made, to give 50 per cent at this initial, trial visit. While the gases are being delivered the administrator must maintain a steady patter of conversation designed to give the patient confidence that he is safe and has control of his situation, by being able to carry on a rational conversation with the administrator. The dentist repeats to the patient that he will have a sense of well being, feel a warm glow pervade his body, and may have a sensation of tingling in his limbs and perhaps his lips. At the trial visit the level of nitrous oxide should not exceed 50 per cent. After this point, 100 per cent oxygen should be administered for three minutes and then the patient allowed to sit up for a few minutes before standing up, under the supervision of the administrator. The patient can be allowed to go home after 15 minutes, if accompanied by a responsible adult and instructed not to drive a car or operate machinery for 12 hours.

At the next visit when conservative dentistry is to be carried out, the process is repeated to the optimal point indicated by the trial visit, before dental work is begun. The process of increasing the nitrous oxide percentage can be shortened. For example, an operator may begin with 10 per cent nitrous oxide instead of 100 per cent oxygen and proceed from that point. If the optimal stage is exceeded, the patient will not be able to co-operate or to open his mouth, and may even lose consciousness. If this occurs, the situation can readily be resolved by decreasing the nitrous oxide percentage by 10–15 per cent. This will produce satisfactory results in 20 seconds or so. It should be expected that ideal operating conditions are obtained with around 50 per cent nitrous oxide though some patients will require more, up to 70 per cent, and others will tolerate treatment with much smaller percentages. Dr Langa himself suggests that some patients can be treated successfully with as little as 15 per cent nitrous oxide.

It is important to ensure that there is no leak of gases or entrainment of air to dilute the nitrous oxide, and that the reservoir bag is not allowed to collapse — this would make inspiration of gases by the patient difficult or impossible — or to become over distended by too high a flow of gases. The average adult has a minute volume of around six litres per minute and a flow rate about this level or slightly above will be required. Advocates of this system of 'Relative Analgesia' — notably Graham J. Roberts of the Royal Dental Hospital who developed basically the technique described here — find that about half of their patients require a local anaesthetic as well as the inhaled nitrous oxide, certainly if extractions are to be accomplished successfully. This injection, often uncomfortable in the conscious patient, can be performed readily under the influence of the nitrous oxide.

The patient must not lie on the dental chair with his legs or ankles crossed during the administration lest this interferes with circulation in the lower limbs. Similarly, care in positioning the arms must be taken in case pressure, of which the patient is unaware because of his treatment, is exerted on nerves or arteries by the chair arms. The gas cylinders must be checked before the administration begins and someone familiar with the procedure must be free to turn on a fresh cylinder should this be required during the treatment. Using the recommended 'Relative Analgesia' machines, the two Quantiflex machines or the McKesson RA/GA apparatus, the nitrous oxide will not flow if the oxygen supply fails; thus the patient would then breathe air and the analgesia would be lost. The dentist should ensure for his own benefit that he is not left alone with the patient and unchaperoned during the treatment of female patients.

It is relevant to the discussion of 'Relative Analgesia' that Guedel's 'First stage of anaesthesia – Analgesia' should be mentioned. More recent studies particularly by G. D. Parbrook of Glasgow Royal Infirmary (1970), have shown that this stage can be subdivided into three planes which can be obtained clinically by administering increasing percentages of nitrous oxide.

Plane 1.
Moderate sedation and analgesia produced by inhaling 5–25 per cent nitrous oxide in oxygen. The patient is mentally relaxed and the circumoral muscles are relaxed enough to allow the dentist access to the mouth for conservation work.

Plane 2.
Psychological detachment and dissociation obtained by inhaling 20–50 per cent nitrous oxide. The patient has a relaxed, faraway look and the rate at which his eyes blink is reduced. There is a tendency to dream and these dreams are most likely to be pleasant. The sedative effect is more pronounced than in the first plane. The patient still responds to questions and commands but at the deeper levels these responses will probably be slowed and speech may be slightly slurred. Tingling of the limb extremities and the lips may be prominent. Amnesia for events occurring during this plane may occur. While the patient is in this plane he is able to keep his mouth wide open for the dentist to work freely and the gag reflex is obtunded.

Plane 3.
Almost total analgesia induced by inhaling 50–70 per cent nitrous oxide. Amnesia is very common. The patient at some stage will almost certainly lose his ability to keep his mouth open and co-operation will be lost. If this point is reached during the administration of 'Relative Analgesia', co-operation can be re-established in twenty

seconds or so when the nitrous oxide level is reduced by 10–15 per cent. If this is not done it will be quite impossible to continue treatment. For this reason it should not be necessary or prudent to use any form of mouth prop during treatment.

The cost of administering gases for relative analgesia will depend on various factors particularly the size of cylinders used— the larger ones are more economical than the smaller ones. The author has calculated that, without including rental charges for the cylinders, using the large M/A size cylinders holding 1900 gallons (8550 litres) of nitrous oxide or 650 gallons (2040 litres) of oxygen, the cost of having a constant flow rate of 4 litres per minute of nitrous oxide along with 4 litres per minute of oxygen is in the region of 55p per half hour, at the prices quoted early in 1979.

The practice of using 'Relative Analgesia' which necessitates the administration of nitrous oxide for long periods raises the question of atmospheric pollution in the surgery premises by low concentrations of nitrous oxide. The extent to which the technique is used will decide the extent of the precautionary measures required. If its use is only occasional then probably all that is required is good room ventilation. If its use is very considerable then a special system designed to vent the waste gas out of the working environment is probably required. At any rate it would be prudent, in any case, for pregnant members of staff not to be present during and soon after a period of possible atmospheric pollution.

At the conclusion of the conservation work and the administration of the gases the patient should be ready to leave the surgery premises within a short time— fifteen minutes or so. It is wise to insist that he be accompanied home by a responsible adult and not permitted to drive a vehicle or operate machinery for twelve hours. Pre-operative preparation should be the same as for a full general anaesthetic — no food or drink for a minimum of four hours and prior to that period food should be light and readily digestible.

If the advice offered for the administration of relative analgesia by the administration of nitrous oxide–oxygen mixtures is followed there should be no excuse for patients refusing dental treatment because of fear of painful stimuli or injections. It should not be necessary to supplement anaesthesia with local anaesthesia but if the dentist chooses to do so so this can readily be done. Without the local anaesthetic the patient should have no painful stimuli and should be able to tolerate otherwise painful manipulations on his teeth. There seems no reason at all why 'Relative Analgesia' should not revolutionise conservative dental treatment in the United Kingdom. It is eminently suitable for children but one must be patient enough and persuasive enough to encourage them to try the system. The author has even heard reports of children being very enthusiastic about their 'Relative Analgesia' sessions and expressing an eager desire for a return visit for the 'happy air'.

8

Economics of dental anaesthesia

While the author appreciates the near futility, because of frequent price increases, of introducing the question of equipment and drug costs it is thought that the dentist or anaesthetist about to equip himself for dental anaesthesia ought to have some idea of the costs involved. It must be appreciated that these prices quoted are approximate only and are those currently in force early in 1979.

Anaesthetic machines
The total cost, at the moment of writing early in 1979, of Quantiflex machines varies between £650 and £750. The M.D.M. apparatus is slightly dearer than the R.A. model. The cost varies according to which stand is required for the head; the stand which carries small cylinders being dearer than the one for use with piped gases. The head may be wall mounted if so desired and this would be less expensive than a mobile stand but would severely restrict its use to one surgery.

The McKesson Simplor apparatus, with stand, costs almost £850. The RA/GA models are less expensive around £585. Conversion units for the earlier Simplor models to enable the anaesthetist to see how much oxygen is contained in the cylinders is around £128, as stated earlier.

The small Boyle apparatus, the International, varies in price depending upon whether it carries cylinders only, and how many, or whether it has pipeline inlets as well. The price range is £784 to £1172.

Vaporisers
The Penlon OMV 50 Halothane vaporiser is quoted about £146, while the Cyprane portable drawover vaporiser is slightly cheaper, around £135. Goldman vaporisers cost about £68 each from BOC Ltd.

Sundry equipment

Oronasal dental inhaler	£27.50
East Scavenging Valve	£37.00
Ferguson Gag (adult)	£12.00

Doyen Gag (adult)	£21 00
Devonshire Dental Prop	£ 2.34
McKesson Dental Prop	£ 2.00
Nasopharyngeal tubes	£ 2.02
Paul's Tubing per metre	£ 0.27
Clear Tape 2.5 cm wide	£ 0.50
Cardiff Aldasorber	£ 4.50
Disposable Syringes – 2 ml	£ 0.045
5 ml	£ 0.07
10 ml	£ 0.08
20 ml	£ 0.115
Needles	£ 0.023 average
Mediswabs	£ 6.12 per 1000

The Syringe and Needle prices are those referrable to hospital bulk purchase. Syringes obtained through other sources may be marginally more expensive.

Drugs
The following is a typical list of drugs required at some time or other by the dental anaesthetist. Some drugs are used regularly while others are only required for use in emergency.

Thiopentone 2.5 gm multidose pack	£1.37
Methohexitone 2.5 gm multidose pack	£4.69
Sterile Water 100 ml	£1.05
Suxamethonium multidose 500 mg/10 ml	£0.96
Halothane 250 ml	£8.19
Trilene 500 ml	£2.00
Hydrocortisone 100 mg with 2 ml water	£0.85
Aminophylline 250 mg in 10 ml	£0.13
Vasoxine injection (methoxamine) 20 mgm	£0.26
Atropine 0.5 mg ampoule	£0.14
K.Y. Jelly 42 gm	£0.39
2% Lignocaine 5 ml	£0.14

It should be noted that all these prices, except those for methohexitone and sterile water, and halothane, are obtained from a hospital pharmacy department and are consequently related to bulk contract prices obtained by a hospital. Small quantity purchases through a private pharmacist would be marginally higher, though probably subject to a professional discount.

In addition to the capital outlay on apparatus the dental anaesthetist has to bear a considerable amount of running costs. These are first of all for halothane and anaesthetic gases. Depending on which firm the halothane is bought from and on how many bottles are purchased at one time, the 250 ml bottle of halothane costs about £8.19. In the author's experience a bottle of this size will be sufficient to anaesthetise 65–70 patients — that is, patients who are given a simple nitrous oxide, oxygen and halothane anaesthetic plus those given an intravenous induction in whom halothane is used as an adjuvant. The cost per patient is therefore 11.5–12.5p.

It is difficult to assess accurately the cost of the gases per patient but the author has found that the total cost of nitrous oxide and oxygen plus the additional costs of delivery, rental of cylinders and V.A.T. amount to between 5 per cent and 9 per cent of the total anaesthetic fees obtained.

For intravenous work we have to consider the cost of disposable syringes and needles, the methohexitone and the sterile water. The cost of a 2.5 g bottle of 'Brietal' is £4.69, sterile water costs about £1.05 per 100 ml, so the cost of making up a 2.5 per cent solution of methohexitone is £5.74. To this is added the cost of a 5 ml ampoule of 2 per cent Lignocaine — 14p, making £5.88 in all. If a 1 per cent solution is used the cost rises to £7.46. Over a large series of cases the author finds that each bottle will be sufficient for 26 doses. This means that each dose on average costs 23p when a 2.5 per cent solution is used and 29p when the 1 per cent solution is used. When one adds the cost of syringes and needles these figures rise to 32p for the 2.5 per cent solution and 42.5p for the 1 per cent solution.

It is worth setting these costs in context against the current general anaesthetic fees paid by the Dental Estimates Board which range from £2.50 when one to three teeth are extracted to £5.50 when over 20 teeth are extracted, the latter being a comparatively rare occurrence. In certain circumstances — where the surgical condition being treated warrants a special anaesthetic technique or there is a medical condition requiring that the patient be handled with special care because of the increased risk involved in administering a general anaesthetic — the Dental Estimates Board has the power to award a discretionary anaesthetic fee of up to £14.00, though their usual maximum is £11.50. The vast majority of fees, however, fall into the lower two categories, the £2.50 fee and the next one £3.20 for 4–11 teeth. The cost of gases plus halothane for a gaseous induction and maintenance average 30p. If an intravenous induction is used simply with nitrous oxide and oxygen only the average cost is 40p using the 2.5 per cent solution or 46p if a 1 per cent solution is used. These costs rise to 52p and 58p respectively if a halothane adjuvant is used. It is not surprising therefore to find these fees severely criticised by the professions when we find that the cost of anaesthetic agents can cost anything from 12 per cent to 23 per cent of the anaesthetic fee, even without taking account of the capital outlay on anaesthetic apparatus. It is a good thing that many dental anaesthetists can find some 'job satisfaction' to compensate them for their efforts. Without it the National Health Service could find itself short of dental anaesthetists everywhere.

REFERENCES

Al-Khishali, T., Padfield, A., Parks, E. R. and Thornton, J. A. (1978) Cardio-respiratory effects of nitrous oxide: oxygen: halothane anaesthesia administered to dental out-patients in the upright position. *Anaesthesia*, 33(2), 187.

Allen, G. D., Gehrig, J. D. and Tolas, A. G. (1969) Evaluation of demand-flow anaesthetic machines in dental practice. *Journal of the American Dental Association*, 78, 99.

Bourne, J. G. (1957) Supine position — fainting and cerebral damage. *Lancet*, 2, 499.

Committee of safety in medicine. (Feb. 1978.) Current problems.

Courville, C. B. (1936) Asphyxia as a consequence of nitrous oxide anaesthesia. *Medicine*, 15, 129.

Goldman, V. (1958) Deaths under anaesthesia in the dental surgery. *British Dental Journal*, 105, 160.

Guedel, A. E. (1951) *Inhalation Anaesthesia*, 2nd edition. New York: Macmillan.

Heath, J. R., Anderson, M. M. and Nunn, J. F. (1973) Performance of the Quantiflex Monitored Dial Mixer. *British Journal of Anaesthesia*, 45, 216.

Langa, H. (1976) *Relative Analgesia in Dental Practice — Inhalation Analgesia and Sedation with Nitrous Oxide*. London: W. B. Saunders Company.

Nainby-Luxmoore, R. C. (1967) Some hazards of dental machines: the report of a survey. *Anaesthesia*, 22, 545.

Parbrook, G. D. (1970) The levels of nitrous oxide analgesia. *General Anaesthesia for Dental Surgery*, ed. Hunter, A. R. and Bush, G. H. Altringcham: John Sherrat.

Wise, C. C., Robinson, J. S., Heath, M. J. and Tomlin, P. J. (1969) Physiological responses to intermittent methohexitone for conservative dentistry. *British Medical Journal* 2, 540–543.

Index